CW00550745

SEX POSITIONS

THE BEST SEX GUIDE FOR COUPLES.

FIND OUT SECRET TIPS TO INCREASE LIBIDO, UNLOCK POWERFUL ORGASMS, AND DISCOVER YOUR SEXUAL ENERGY

Amanda Shein

TABLE OF CONTENTS:

Introduction

Welcome to Sex Positions and thank you for purchasing. I will take you on a journey of exploration. Read this book with an open mind, and you will learn a myriad of ways to take your sex life to the next level as a couple. Through reading this book, you will learn new techniques and skills like new sex positions and how best to lead a woman to orgasm. You will also learn other types of skills such as how to increase intimacy and how to get into the mood. This book touches on every aspect of sex from beginning to end and will allow you to hone your sex skills in order to impress your partner and strengthen your relationship. If you have ever wondered what else you can do to improve your sex life, or what might be missing, this book will show you all of that and more. By reading this book, even the sections that you may think you know already, you will be able to brush up on things you are familiar with, which is always a good thing.

There are some things to keep in mind when it comes to sex, and in this introduction, we will cover these first before diving in. The first thing we are going to discuss are the differences to keep in mind when having sex in a relationship versus casual sex. For some of you, relationship sex may be new, or it may be a while since you have been in a relationship. For this reason, we are going to go over some things that you should note when you enter a relationship. Communication is the key to a good relationship, sex aside. When it comes to sex, communication is key there, as well. This is especially true when in a long-term relationship. When having casual sex, communication is helpful since then you can figure out what the person likes and dislikes, but oftentimes it takes trial and error to find out how to please that person. Likely by the time you figure out exactly how to do so, you have moved onto the next person. When having sex in a relationship, you have much more time to talk about sex and find out what that person likes and dislikes. You may even feel more pressure to please them since you value their feelings and want to make them feel good. Being able to communicate during sex is great for a relationship because you can be learning in the moment. When you are learning in the moment, you know exactly what the person is referring to instead of having to recall it later. This does not have to happen like a visit to the doctor where they ask you "does this hurt?" you can indicate to each other what you like by telling them that "this feels good" or "keep going" without ruining the sensual mood. Being able to do this will help both of you to be pleased in the long-term.

The other reason that communication is so essential in a relationship sex is that people's likes and needs change over time. If you have been with someone for six years, they may have developed new preferences in terms of their pleasure. Being able to communicate this will allow for continued pleasure no matter how long you are together. Aside from changing needs, you and your partner want to keep sex interesting. When you are having casual sex, you will meet up once or twice and do whatever feels good that day. When you are in a relationship, you will likely develop somewhat of a routine that you know gives you both pleasure every time. This can become dull after a while, so being able to communicate about what you both would like to try will help to keep your sex life new and fresh. It is rare that you will talk about sex and new things that you would like to try in the bedroom with a one-night stand, but when in a relationship having talks about sex outside of the bedroom in times when you aren't horny will keep you both informed about where the other person stands when it comes to sex.

By taking the above into consideration, you will be well on your way to having a fulfilling and pleasurable sex life no matter how long you have been in a relationship for. A dull sex life is not inevitable, and by maintaining the lines of communication in your relationship, you will be able to keep yourselves happy and fulfilled. In addition to being fulfilled sexually, this will keep you both fulfilled in your relationship as a whole. A good sex life is important to having a close and healthy relationship. Prioritizing this will lead to a better overall relationship. Sex is hard to talk about, so being able to do this will strengthen your bond overall.

One final tip on this topic is to be open-minded when discussing these things with your partner. It may be hard for them to open up to you about things that they want to try or how they want you to please

—

them. Being open-minded and non-judgmental will help them to feel safe and secure in this territory. This goes for all genders. Men will often not voice their insecurities when it comes to sex, but this does not mean they don't have them. By being open and listening to their desires, they will feel safe opening up to you over and over again. Getting comfortable with these types of dialogues can take time, so have patience with yourself and your partner, and most of all, enjoy!

Before Sex

Foreplay

Foreplay is an activity at the beginning of a sexual encounter that aims at building sexual arousal and brings orgasm in preparation for sexual intercourse. It is a crucial part of sexual experience and acts as a determinant of satisfaction.

Importance of Foreplay

· Biological: Couples need to indulge in foreplay for it causes erection of both the penis and the clitoris. An erection is crucial for it enhances penetration and orgasm among women. Therefore, it creates the best conditions for biological activity. Besides, foreplay elicits wetness making penetration easier for the couples. Lack of vaginal wetness is associated with painful intercourse and bleeding.

· Psychological: Foreplay is known to instill a feeling of care and security among couples. Failure to make foreplay makes your partner feel neglected and denied emotional assurance. The concern of your partner's feeling before sex serves as an indicator that you are not in for selfish gains but mutual pleasure.

Types of Foreplay

Foreplay is the ultimate time to build tension and sexual chemistry between partners. If you lack mind-blowing sex, you should focus on foreplay. Notably, sex is more realistic and complex than television and movies show. For that reason, when you intimately touch, smell, hear, and taste your partner, they would argue it as better than penetration.

The following are types of foreplay that you should work before sex.

1. Sexy Materials: You could practice foreplay at any time and manner. You do not have to be naked to engage in foreplay. When at

home or work you may watch a sexy movie or read sexy materials. These materials could help you maintain orgasm for hours.

2. Undressing: If you usually take off your clothes before sex, then you might be missing a lot of foreplay. Having your fingers hold your partner's outfits and graze on their body as you undress them is highly stimulating and arousing. Depending on how sensitive they are, you might witness them getting goosebumps.

3. Vagina stroking: It involves how you put your hands down there and caressing on her pants and panties. Light strokes on the region make her wet and stimulated for sex.

4. Kisses and caressing: Though kisses do not lead to sex, most sexual activities involve kisses and touching. As part of foreplay, kisses should start slow and intensify gradually. Kisses on the neck and boobs are most arousing for women.

5. Boob Action: Teases made on their breasts arouse women. Therefore, you should suck, kiss and rub them, taking advantage of the sensitive nerve ending in the nipples. The foreplay should be done with moderation to avoid hurting your partner.

6. Dry Hump: It involves gently grinding on your partner. It can happen when naked to show how moody you are. The foreplay plays a significant role in heating the moment for intercourse.

7. Breathing: Yes, you are right; your breath arouses and stimulates your partner, especially when done on sensitive areas such as genitals and neck. In this case, bad breath would be counterproductive.

8. Hands-On: Your hands are a piece of efficient equipment when it comes to foreplay. You should use them to grab your partner's breasts, rub their hair, and thighs. In short, use your hands to explore your partner's body unless they say no.

9. Oral: If you are okay in giving oral, you should incorporate it into your foreplay routine. Be a little bit gentle by teasing, sucking, and licking the clitoris and allowing time.

10. Labia love: As a highly ignored part, labia have numerous nerve endings that are perfect for arousal and stimulation. You can massage them slowly or hold them gently between fingers.

11. Ass: If you and your partner are into stimulation through the anus, then you should try it out effectively. The most ignored nerve endings in the anus cause sexual stimulation, especially if gently licked.

12. Multitask: You may incorporate all of these techniques and concurrently make different moves. With the perfect combination, you make your partner fantasized with enjoyable sexual stimulation

How Do I Give Mind-Blowing Foreplay?

The list of foreplay techniques proves that the activity is a real deal when it comes to sexual arousal. Similarly, mastering the best and most applicable to your partner is a significant step towards sexual satisfaction. You may learn the best technique, but wrong application of foreplay may be counterproductive to both partners. For that reason, it is advisable to understand the following steps when going for foreplay.

- Relax: Although partners have different timeframes to achieve orgasm, it may take about 3 minutes and twenty minutes for men and women respectively. So, you should take your time and allow time to climax.

- Make it gradual: You should start the foreplay with the areas away from the genitals with slow stimulation. With hot breaths, kisses, stroking, you are sure to achieve orgasm once you hit the spot.

- Caress gently: You should make progressive touches on the less apparent spots of your partner's body, such as buttocks and inner thighs. You should delight the nipples with light feathery touches. In the same way, you should gradually approach the genitals from the outer layers as you move inner.

· Adjust Stimulation: An ongoing touch on nerve endings reduces their sensitivity. Therefore, you should vary strokes from light to strong and move from one spot to another.

· Seek Feedback: Most partners feel shy, asking for what they want in foreplay. However, they appreciate it when asked if they enjoy the foreplay. With questions like "How does it feel?" there is good communication and willingness to please a partner. The practice promotes intimacy and enjoyable sex.

· Practice: You should indulge in foreplay without penetration to know your partner and lead them to repeat orgasms. Continued engagement in other forms of sexual interaction acts as an eye-opener in your sexual horizons.

Sex may hurt if your partner is not ready. Foreplay acts as a preparation for enjoyable sexual intercourse. Ensure that you apply the foreplay that best fits you to avoid accidents and incidents.

Erotic Massage

Our bodies have tremendous capabilities to experience pleasure through the five ordinary senses. Above all, the sense of touch is explored to attain exquisite joy, especially in intimacy. If you are in a loving relationship, erotic massage is a means you could use to stimulate each other. Chiefly, touch, and massage is a powerful tool for sexual foreplay. The erotogenic aspect of the human body aids in receiving the tactile massages of desire, love, and tenderness. At the same time, the soul and emotions become nourished.

Benefits of Erotic Massage

Whether you are giving or receiving the massage, you should dissolve into your space and learn to do it without criticism. That way, you rest assured to experience the following benefits from the feeling of touch.

1. Facilitates orgasm: Erotic massages are mostly meant to cause sexual stimulation. As a result, men experience erection while women get wet and moody. These are body responses to allow for perfect intercourse.

2. Enhances Relationships: If you would like to see your relationship blossom, then you need to incorporate erotic massage in your foreplay. The practice requires you to be emotionally open and conscious. Consequently, you develop a mutual connection that promotes your relationship.

3. Relieves anxiety: Your body has endorphin that allows muscle relaxation after the massage. The relaxation helps reduce stress and anxiety, making it a perfect after-work must do.

4. Fights Inflammation: Erotic massage is ideal in improving your muscle health and joints. It relaxes and stimulates aching and overworked muscles. Your body becomes flexible and refreshed to proceed with the daily routine.

5. Tone the Skin: Erotic massage cleanses your skin by rubbing it gently and unblocking pores. You remain clean as you wipe unwanted layers. Incorporation of massage oil plays a significant role in reviving the natural tone of your skin.

6. Improves Blood Circulation: During the massage, the blood flows throughout the body to meet the threshold for sexual stimulation. The heart pumps in moderation as the relaxation enhances circulation.

7. Relaxes Muscles: As you receive the message, your body experiences gentle and frequent muscle contractions. The process of compressing the muscles is vital in correcting rigid tendons.

8. Regulates Hormones: Massages are known to cause pleasure and stimulation. Specifically, erotic massage helps in boosting your moods and urge. Further, the massage improves your immune system, thus improving the ability to fight infections.

What You Need

Before indulging in the act, itself, you should first recall a previous massage session. Create an atmosphere that surpasses what you experienced. In most cases, couples would need to take a warm shower to help relax muscles. The following preparations are crucial in making your room a haven of seduction.

- Get Rid of Distractions: The most crucial thing about erotic massage is that it works miracles in a quiet and peaceful place. Therefore, you should settle and focused on the activity while avoiding interruptions. Notably, the requirement includes all sorts of distractions, whether physical or psychological.

- Lighting: Erotic massage is perfect when done in relatively dim light to create an ethereal atmosphere. For that reason, you should set sources of dim light such as candles to make it warm and cozy. You should apply proper caution as you may be prone to burns.

- Fragrance: Scents play a significant role in influencing a person's moods and memories. The application of essential oils and incense sticks provide a therapeutic and pleasant fragrance.

- Music: Music is also an important part, especially if it is suitable for erotic massage. It should create a spa atmosphere and should even flow in a sexual and soothing mood.

- Temperature: While most couples may prefer a naked erotic massage, the room temperature should be regulated accordingly. You may use a warm sheet to keep your partner comfortable during the massage. Room temperature would be preferable but might be subject to change depending on your adaptation.

How Is It Done?

You should start with gentle touches as you build comfort and confidence with the process. Your partner should help you in deciding whether to start with the hands or feet. The fact that sensual massage acts as foreplay means that you should feel free to seduce your partner. Therefore, you are required to increase physical contact for great feelings of intimacy. Feel free to massage the whole body and pay close attention to nerve endings. Application of techniques serves as a powerful gift that is pleasurable, intimate, and demonstrates selflessness.

Types of Erotic Massage

In addition to releasing stress and tension, erotic massage can also help you focus on the pleasurable sensation. In most cases, these forms of massage end up in ejaculation or orgasms.

1.   Soapy Massage: It starts in the shower when naked couples rub soap onto one another. The soap aids in giving a smooth massage as well as cleaning them for further massage or sex.

2.   Duo Massage: It mostly involves two people giving and receiving luxurious massage. Both the giver and the receiver apply oil on their bodies for a perfect body to body massage.

3.   Prostate Massage: This form of massage aims at stimulating the prostate glands mostly believed to be a man's emotional, sacred, and sexual spot. Stimulated prostate releases psychological and physical pressure that creates an intense experience.

4.   Lingam Massage: It involves honoring the stimulation and sensations of the penis through massage. It includes gentle touches on the testicles, shaft, and the perineum. It is meant to create sensual stimulation from a thorough genital massage.

5.   Yoni Massage: Such as the lingam, Yoni involves loving, respecting, and honoring vaginal stimulation through massage. A relaxed yoni

massage helps create acceptance of the sexual feelings experienced. This type of erotic massage is beneficial, especially if you want to release sexual issues such as sexual pain and anorgasmia. It is known to build trust and respect in relationships.

Erotic massage is vital in your foreplay, for it allows you to influence your partner's sexual desires. You develop a mutual concept when you exercise different forms of erotic massage. However, you should be careful and deliberate not to mistake a tickle for a massage.

Learning to Make Love

As a couple, you may have similar desires and wants, but the sequence required may differ. In most cases, men are known to take less time to achieve sexual stimulation as compared to women. If you are inexperienced in making love or seem to be unskilled, you need to understand what making love entails. How you approach your partner as well as the way you handle the situation plays a significant role in achieving orgasm. It would be advisable to research what you could be doing wrong if your partner complains of sexual dissatisfaction. Similarly, you could explore additional information on ways to make your lovemaking livelier and more enjoyable. The following detailed steps to step guide will help you on how you could be a pro in making love.

1.   Nurture your self-esteem: Appreciating your personality and character is the initial point where you develop an excellent reflection about yourself. You should explore your thoughts honestly and openly to identify the aspect that could be hindering you from attaining your full potential. Similarly, you realize your strengths and weaknesses are making it easier to gauge your potential and select tasks. This way, you will be able to relieve yourself of the things that cannot be changed as well as those that are from the past. Notably, this process requires ample time to internalize the steps you need to take to get rid of negative interactions that always drag you behind. It may even entail adjusting your environment and finding time to do what you enjoy.

The critical aspect of improving your self-esteem is embracing change. As it may be difficult in the initial stage, you need to be patient and perseverant to achieve the benefits of being a confident, healthier, and happier person.

2. Improve Your Lifestyle: After developing high self-esteem and making the right moves to understand yourself, you remain qualified to build a healthy love life. As you explore those various aspects that will offer guidance on your dating life, you need to keep on developing your confidence and selecting a reasonable target. You will realize that making love involves flirting, teasing, and providing compliments as you aim to take your partner to the bed. Developing your intimacy skills will play a vital role in arousing your mind, which then makes you anticipate a gentle touch and intimacy. Besides, you should note that how you present yourself is an excellent determinant of the partner you win and their perception about you. Therefore, you must get a life and begin to make natural moves of seduction and arousal.

3. Understand What It Is to Make Love: This is an essential part of making love for you might mistake making love for sex. If you do not see any difference, then you might not have experienced it. Sex is familiar to everyone and involves biomechanical and instinctive intercourse. On the contrary, lovemaking is all about the art of sensual and slow romance. Lovemaking is meant to create a connection between partners. The motivation for lovemaking differs from that of sex. Lovemaking is a complex act of expressing love and satisfying your partner. It is an activity where your body, soul, and mind are equally involved in getting to each other's heart. The openness associated with lovemaking allows all forms of communication, leaving no room for wandering. Lovemaking starts long before intercourse and may continue after that. For that reason, you should consider lovemaking as an emotional activity but not just undressing and romping on the bed.

4. Pick Perfect Location: Lovemaking should happen in a place where you feel comfortable and undistracted. Therefore, you should ensure that the site you choose for lovemaking is romantic. If you would like

to make it more personal, you could select a comfortable room in your house where you are aware of the environment. Be creative while choosing your location and consider aspects such as weather and your partner's preference. Also, the temperature of your preferred location should be in line with the activity ahead as too warm or cold could make it a mess. Remember to put away all forms of distractions to avoid losing the true meaning of making love.

5. Set the Mood: If it is your first time to make love, you need to be sure and comfortable about what you are about to do. Ensure that you are aware of what is about to happen and decide on what outcomes you expect. Similarly, make the ambiance conducive and appropriate for lovemaking. When you are in for it avoid being silly or making tasteless jokes thinking that your partner likes it. Instead, settle on a romantic atmosphere where everything you do aims at soothing them and causing sexual stimulation. With this course, your partner will feel appreciated, safe, and cherished through cuddling and gentle touches. Setting the mood may also involve sexy details such as dirty words, music, movies, dim light, and lingerie. When the attitude is right, you will tell from the responses you get from your partner as well as your body reaction.

Different Type of Sex and Best Positions

Sensual positions

Being rough and spontaneous in the bedroom certainly has a time and a place, but sometimes you want to slow it all down and really become intimate with your partner. Sex does not always need to be hard and fast in order for it to be great, and we want to highlight some of the absolute best sensual positions that are still guaranteed to have you both reaching the peak of pleasure.

All of these positions incorporate similar elements that make them more romantic, more intimate, and more sensual. Things like being faced to face, having a high degree of closeness, or allowing for more touching, all are a part of what makes these more pleasing.

Spooning

What is the position?

The king of the sensual positions, Spooning allows for extreme closeness and intimacy due to the comforting position and classic cuddling that it brings to mind. Just like when it is used in a non-sexual way, this position begins with the woman lying on her side, and the man lying on his side behind her. From here he will enter from behind, wrapping an arm around her waist and kissing against her neck. The man's hands are very free in this position, so he is able to roam around, and the angle allows for you to go nice and slow in order to really up the romance.

What makes this position worth trying?

This position truly feels like you are cuddling with your partner, so it can feel very comforting and relaxing. Not only is it very positive mentally, but physically it can lead to serious pleasure as the way the woman's legs will typically lay makes for a tighter vaginal opening. The angle can make G-Spot contact easier, and the woman also has the ability to reach down and play with her clitoris. Overall, this is a fantastic position that many people put in their top favorite lists.

How to enhance the position?

Like with most positions, there are countless variations that people like to use to either make the position even more intimate, or to switch up the angle and sensations. Given that the standard variation lacks that face to face contact, we will include some variations that actually allow for that to happen, in order to make everything a lot more sensual.

•   Bent Spoon – This position uses a bit of a bend in body shape in order to create some distance and make it possible for the woman to turn back and look at her man. From the standard position, the woman will need to move her upper body forward, away from the man, so that she creates space between the partners. From here, she will twist her upper body slightly, and look back so that she is now face to face with the man. While this variation may not change up the sensation or angle of penetration, is does go a long way in making the partners feel more connected. Being able to stare into your partner's eyes while they slow penetrate you makes this one of the top choices for sensual positions.

•   Wrapped Spoon – This variation will change up the angle as well as the sensation, as it involves the woman having her legs wider open, which will open up the vagina. Keeping the same pose as with the standard variation, the woman will now lift her top leg and place it behind the man's legs. For couples that may struggle with rear entry positions, this can make it significantly easier as the woman is now more accessible to the man. The does not change the intimacy factor, however, as your bodies are still tightly pressed against each other, and it actually can feel more intimate since your legs are now entwined with one another.

•   Crossed Spoon – The most drastic variation from the one's we've discussed so far; this actually makes it, so the partners are no longer pressed against one another. If you are thinking that this will remove the sensual nature of spooning, think again! With the man still laying on his side as normal, the woman will now position herself to the side of the man, with her head facing away from him and her legs place over top of his body. Inching closer, she will scoot forward until she is against his pelvis and he will enter from this angle. What makes this variation so good is that it involves face to face contact without the need to twist and bend. You will be looking directly into each other's eyes, and you can hold hands as your partner thrusts into you.

Saint

What is the position?

Make your partner feel like the angel they are, with this intimate and close-contact position. Not only is this position extremely sensual, but it also offers up a significant number of variations in order to make it sexier, spicier, and even more romantic. For the standard position, you will need to have the man kneeling down, with his buttocks placed against the back of his feet. The woman will now straddle him, legs on either side, feet planted firmly on the ground behind the man. Your bodies should be pressed together, face to face, and the man will have his arms wrapped around the woman while her hands are against his chest. To make this more comfortable, have the man place a pillow under his knees so that they aren't pressing into the hard ground, and instead he can simply focus on the pleasure.

What makes this position worth trying?

This is a very intimate position, as both partners are pressed together, and their faces are only inches apart. On top of that, this position offers a lot of variation, as well as great penetration even in the standard pose. The man is able to thrust fairly easily, while still having his hands free to roam around his partner's body. As for the woman, she is able to bounce on her partner if she so chooses, meaning that each person can take turns with who is doing the majority of the work.

How to enhance the position?

As we said above, this position has more variations than we could possibly include in this book, so we are going to look at some of the more common and popular ones in order to highlight how you can go about adjusting this position in order to meet your personal needs. Some of those variations include:

•   Kneeling Saint – For women who want to play a more active role and be able to have control over depth and speed, the Kneeling

Saint is the perfect variation to try. Instead of sitting on her man and putting her feet behind him, the woman will now kneel as well, with her knees on either side of the man's knees. This variation maintains all of the intimacy associated with the original, and instead the only difference it truly makes is that it allows for the woman to bounce up and down more easily.

•   Folded Saint – Bringing her legs up off of the ground, this variation has the woman placing her legs over her man's shoulders, while he still remains in the same kneeling position. This may seem like a minor change, but it actually shifts the angle from which the man enters, making it better suited for a distinct grinding motion rather than the standard thrusting usually seen. Grinding against the woman can be very pleasurable for both people involved, and it is sure to bring about new sensations, since most people typically focus on just the in and out motion during sex.

•   Wrapped Saint – With the Wrapped Saint, the woman will wrap her legs around her partner's waist and then cross them behind him. This can up the intimacy as it feels closer and tighter than other variations, almost as if the woman is hugging him during sex. The man can also alter his position as well, and instead of staying kneeling, he can instead sit on his buttocks cross legged. Almost like a meditative pose, this added variation will make thrusting a bit more difficult, but it will up the closeness and feel so much more sensual than other positions.

Spicy positions

•   Missionary

Missionary position is that classic that you may think you are tired of. It may be the position that you began with and stuck to for many years in your early sexual days. It gets a bad reputation as the vanilla position that is only for prudes. Missionary though does not have to be known as the tired old high school position. A missionary position can actually be very very hot and intense if you make it so!

•   Doggy Style

The doggy style position is a favorite among men and women alike. Both women and men can get intense pleasure from this position because the angles at which their genitals come together creates harmonic pleasure.

- The Hound

If you love the feelings you can get and the overall positioning of Doggy Style, but you miss the closeness and intimacy of good ol' Missionary, The Hound is a position that you will love.

You can transition to this position easily when already having sex in the classic Doggy Style position. While sensually thrusting your penis into your woman from behind her on your knees, lean forward and wrap your body around hers. Continue to move your body in the same way, and you will be able to thrust into her more deeply from here. You can thrust quickly or slowly, deeply or shallowly, depending on how much you want to tease your woman and how much you want her to beg you for more. To pleasure her even more, reach your arm around to the front of her body and caress her breasts or stimulate her nipples. From here, slide your hand down the front of her body and begin to play with her clitoris, pumping your penis into her all the while.

- Cowgirl

As you probably already know, it is quite a bit harder for a woman to reach an orgasm from penetration than it is for a man. A woman can have two different types of orgasms, one from stimulating the clitoris and a different one from penetrating, hitting the G-spot. This could be why your girlfriend can reach an orgasm from oral or when you play with her clitoris but has trouble actually reaching the same level when you are having penetrative sex. In many positions, the G-spot is not actually stimulated by the man's penis and this can result in the woman having some pleasure, but not being able to get all the way there.

- Reverse Cowgirl

Reverse Cowgirl is another woman on top position and is beneficial for the woman as there is more likelihood of the female orgasm occurring in this position, just like the regular Cowgirl position. This one is also

20

beneficial for the man because of the view he will have in this position that will make him horny from the get-go.

- 69

69 is a classic position that you have no doubt heard about a number of times. Traditional 69 got its name because both bodies together look like a 69 as one person is facing the other but inverted, just like the number 69.

Oral sex and best sex positions

Oral sex can seem a bit intimidating to some people if they have never participated in it; however, it is actually easier than you think to provide oral pleasure.

Your willingness to try is the number one component. Here again, communication is extremely important. When you can voice to your partner what feels the best it can help guide them on what to do next. If you are very inexperienced you may not know what feels good until it is happening, using your words during any type of sexual play is always encouraged.

One of the key components in ensuring that your lady enjoys oral sex is to be patient with her. You should always start off slow as it builds tension and allows your woman to become extremely aroused. Taking your time is extremely important. Women tend to take more time and need more buildup than men, so patience is definitely a virtue in the realm of oral sex.

Another great tip is don't forget to use your hands. While oral sex, obviously, is going to involve your mouth using your hands at the same time can be truly erotic. Our fingertips can provide a lot of sensation and help to keep things exciting if it is taking a bit of time.

Don't be afraid to ask your female counterpart what it is that she wants. None of us are mind readers and a man will never understand exactly what it feels like for the woman when she receives oral sex. If you are unsure of what you are doing or what exactly it is that she wants simply asking is the best way to go. Some people are afraid to do this because they don't think that it is sexy; However, women much prefer you to ask questions then to simply fumble around.

You must also keep in mind that while the clitoris is an important piece all of your lady's vagina, is extremely important. Taking the time to kiss and caress all areas of her nether regions will certainly get her ready to go. This is another place where your hands should come into play. Taking your time and slowly working all of the sensitive areas of her lower half will help to ensure that she will be able to reach a climax when you provide oral stimulation.

Most women really love the act of being pleased orally so you need to be enthusiastic about it. Sure, for some people it is not going to be their favorite thing but if she's going down on you, you should always return the favor. If your partner feels that you are into the act it will be easier for them to be truly in do it as well. On the other hand, if she doesn't feel that you are excited to be pleasing her orally it will be much more difficult for her to reach climax.

Some people are quite uncomfortable when it comes to receiving oral sex. This can be due to a low level of self-esteem or simply feeling self-conscious about the act that is happening. Communicating with your partner and letting them know that you find them genuinely sexy and that you are excited to please them will help put them in the right state of mind to enjoy all of the oral pleasure you are about to provide them.

You should also be aware that you don't always need to stop right after your partner has an orgasm. Keep in mind there are women that will stop you after one because their clitoris becomes extremely sensitive. However, some women will be more than satisfied to let you keep going. In fact, many women will be able to achieve the second orgasm much more quickly than the first if you continue on.

Now that we've looked at a few things let's talk about the actual process. As noted, you should start off slow and gradually increase the speed. You can also incorporate things like humming. It will provide a different sensation to your female's clitoris and it can be truly amazing. You can work with different vibration speeds that will resonate throughout her entire pelvic area. This is a technique that drives most women wild.

Now that we have looked at some ways you can ensure your female counterpart has a fantastic time during oral stimulation we're going to move on. Making sure that the ladies understand how to take care of their men is equally important. So, let's look at some different ways that women can ensure that they are pleasing their men while providing oral stimulation.

Connection Between Yoga and Sex

Yoga for Advanced Sex Positions

To help with your transition into more advanced sex positions, it is a great idea to practice yoga so that there is less risk of injury and discomfort while allowing your body to move more smoothly into positions that require more physical fitness. Yoga is a great practice even if it is practiced for reasons other than improving your sexual function. It helps you become more aware of your body and teaches you to listen to the physical signs that your body sends you. It also allows you to become more in-tune with your mind so you can control your mental abilities.

The following yoga positions that will be discussed are particularly helpful to females.

- The Happy Baby Pose

This pose is good for strengthening the lower back and gluteus. It also doubles as a great missionary position variation. To achieve this pose, lie on your back and bend your knees up toward your stomach while you exhale. When you inhale, reach to grab the inside of your feet and widen your knees. While pushing your heels upward, flex your feet and pull down with your hands to stretch.

- Child's Pose

This pose helps you become more flexible as it opens up your hips. This pose is also a grounding one as it allows you to focus on resting and practicing breathing techniques which help melt away stress and anxiety. Enter this pose by kneeling on the floor and widening your knees until they are hip width apart. On an exhale, lean forward and place your hands in front of you to stretch out. Allow your upper body to relax between your legs and touch your forehead to the floor. Hold this pose for 30 seconds to a few minutes.

Kama Sutra

It is unlikely that you have never heard of the Kama Sutra before, but you may be unfamiliar with what exactly it is. Some may think of it as simply a book of sex positions, while others may know a bit more of the history and how it came to be. Here will look at the history behind the Kama Sutra, discussing the literal meaning of the words, as well as what it teaches us, and how it is meant to be used. Since the Kama Sutra originated in India, there are also many terms and words used throughout that you may not be familiar with, so we will make sure to breakdown some of the most commonly seen ones and provide their definitions.

With such a rich history behind it, there is so much to learn about the Kama Sutra. It is an expansive work of literature that was created to be more than just a guide on different ways in which you can have sex. Instead, it permeates all aspects of life and brings together both sexual and non-sexual ways in which you interact with a lover, a partner, or a spouse. But what exactly does "Kama Sutra" mean?

Meaning Behind the Name

The word Kama is one that means pleasure but can also be translated as desire or longing. There is a sexual connotation associated with the word, meaning it is more to do with sexual pleasure and desire than with the pleasures of life or desire for material goods, but that doesn't mean that the Kama Sutra as a whole is limited to only sexual pleasure. Sutra, on the other hand, translates to verse or scripture. When you put these words together, you get the translation of "Scripture of Pleasure", but there are many variations on how you can literally translate this.

Delving deeper into the meaning behind the name, the pleasure that is Kama is one that is of all five senses, and this is very important. While many thinks of the Kama Sutra as a sex book, it is actually a book that focuses on pleasing all of the senses and is meant to be a guide on how to live a good life and enjoy yourself. From the physical enjoyment of sex to the pleasure that is derived from being in love, the Kama Sutra is filled with different verses that cover a wide range of different activities and pleasures.

While we did mention that Kama often has a sexual connotation, like with all translations there are different meanings depending on how it is being used. Kama can also be used when referencing love or affection, and in this sense, it is used in a non-sexual way. This is why the Kama Sutra needs to be viewed as a whole, since it was not intended to simply be a sexual book, but more so an erotic manual on life.

We know that the Kama Sutra extends beyond just the physical pleasures, as the book touches on the four different virtues of life. Those four are:

- Dharma – How to live a virtuous life

- Kama – How to enjoy the pleasures of the senses

- Moksha – How to be liberated from the cycle of reincarnation

- Artha – How to gain material wealth

These four virtues are tenants of Hinduism, which is applicable since the Kama Sutra originates in India where Hinduism is one of the predominant religions. This historical context allows us to understand the book better, as we need to approach it from the mindset of the author, who would have most likely been a practicing Hindu. The author saw sexual pleasure as one of the main virtues of life, and it was both a necessary and spiritual pursuit that was important both from a non-sexual and sexual avenue. These virtues are almost instructions on how a person should live in order to be fulfilled both in this life as well as in the afterlife. Regardless of what your personal religion is, all the points are still applicable, as basic human nature dictates that we are all attempting to be the best version of ourselves and to accomplish everything we set out to gain.

Some other words that you may encounter within the Kama Sutra, and their translations, are:

- Devi – Goddess

- Gandharva – A form of marriage in which everyone is consenting to it

- Lingam – Penis

- Nayika – A woman who is desired by someone

- Prahanana – Striking or slapping someone during sex

- Raja – King

- Shlokas – Messages from above that are used to end every chapter of the Kama Sutra

- Vatsala – A married woman who has children

- Vikrant – A brave and beloved man

- Yoni – Vagina

We will try and use as much of the original language as possible, so having a glossary of terms will be beneficial. With that said, however, there will always be translations available throughout so that you can follow along with ease.

So why does the literal meaning of the name even matter?

Well, understanding what an author is trying to convey is important as it allows us to enter the book and adjust our personal views so that we do not bring in our biases and preconceived notions. If you come into the Kama Sutra thinking it should only include some sex positions and nothing more, then you miss out on the richness that is contained within. Likewise, if you ignore the historical significance behind the text, you fail to grasp many of the concepts located within. In order to gain as much as you can from the Kama Sutra, you need to know what the author intended with it, and why they felt the need to create this work of literature.

History of the Kama Sutra

The exact date that the Kama Sutra was written is not known, but estimates place it anywhere between 400 BCE and 300 CE. What we do know, however, is that it was officially compiled and turned into the book that we know today in the 2nd century, otherwise known as 2 CE. This does not mean though that the book has not undergone revisions since then, and some scholars believe that the version we have is actually closely linked to the 3rd century, as some of the references throughout would not have been applicable to the 2nd century. With the text being so old, exact dating is virtually impossible, nevertheless, there is a lot of information we do know about it.

We do know that the text originates from India, although the exact location is unknown. Historians have been able to narrow down the location to somewhere within the north, or northwest, region but beyond that, it is a guess as to where the author was from. As for the author himself, we do know it was written by a man named Vatsyayana Mallanaga, as his name is engraved into the beginning of the text. Who this man was is unclear, but we do have information as to why he wrote the Kama Sutra?

Since it's compilation in the 2nd-3rd century, the Kama Sutra has undergone numerous translations and there are versions in almost every language. It was originally written in Sanskrit, an ancient Indian language, and this is the language that many Hindu scriptures were written in. While some translations are quite accurate, it is important to note that some translators did place their own bias into their work and that can be seen in the discrepancies that were later found. One of the key examples of this was in the 19th century, when the Kama Sutra was translated into English. The translator at that time wanted to ensure that the role of women in the sexual realm was not as prominent, as that was not the culture of the times. In order to maintain that societal understanding of sex and women, the Kama Sutra was altered so that women were significantly downplayed throughout. This has since been corrected, but it is important to be aware of this if you ever decide to pick up a copy for yourself as you want to be sure you are getting a purer translation.

The foundations of the Kama Sutra are rooted within the Vedic Era of literature, which is based on the word Vedas. Vedas were historical texts written in India around this time that dealt with lifestyle and how one should conduct themselves on a daily basis. All works of this time period were verbally passed down, and traditions were later adapted into many of the Hindu beliefs that are now practiced today. In the Vedic Era, there were distinct classes and castes within society, and a lot of that is reflected within the Kama Sutra. Many references are made to those who are in differing classes, and how relationships between individuals of different castes cannot work out. While this type of information is not apparently meaningful in today's culture, it does cross over when we look at socio-economic statuses and how the rich and poor interact even today.

These foundations are incredibly important because they shape the mind frame of the author of the Kama Sutra. Without grasping the history, you cannot possibly grasp what is being discussed, as many of the terms and concepts no longer exist or are practiced currently.

It is with this in mind that we can start to see that the Kama Sutra is a religious text by some accounts. We may not associate sex and religion as being intertwined, but in fact, Vatsyayana saw sex as being a religious experience as well as a requirement to live a proper life. The basis of the entire viewpoint stems from certain religious beliefs, and the foundation for the entire book comes from his personal, religious beliefs. It is a celebration of human sexuality and the most carnal of pleasures, which are gifts from the gods and ultimately a necessity in life.

Philosophy of the Kama Sutra

As we said, we do know a bit about why Vatsyayana wrote the Kama Sutra. Looking at ancient Hindu texts, we know that the four virtues were commonly discussed and written at length about. Many of the texts focused on the two important virtues of Dharma (morality), and Athra (prosperity), while few really delved into the importance of Kama (pleasure). Vatsyayana meditated upon this reality and came to the conclusion that Kama was just as important as all of the other virtues, and so it was only proper to have a guide written solely about how to obtain Kama.

The four virtues can be looked at more as goals that each person much work towards within their lifetime in order to lead a complete and fulfilled life. Within the Kama Sutra, there are many references to the other virtues as they are all tied together and must be achieved in order to succeed. One cannot simply focus on the physical pleasures and ignore the need for morality or prosperity, so you may notice throughout that sex and morality are often combined, as well as sex and finding a partner that brings about monetary prosperity.

- The Widely Open Position

The Widely Open Position begins with the woman laying down on her back. She should keep her head low and against the bed, while she raises up her hips so that they are higher than her head. Keeping her knees bent, her feet should not touch the ground, and instead, her knees should touch against the man's upper back. This position is designed to allow for the yoni to widen. Her partner should be kneeling between her legs, raised up so that he can meet her with his lingam. Her buttocks and lower back should rest comfortably upon his knees, while his hands grasp her sides. To bring her up higher, he may grasp on to her buttocks and raise her lower half to meet him. To increase the deepness of penetration, the woman should clasp on to the man's ankles, so that she may pull herself more tightly towards him.

This position is great for women who are with more well-endowed men, as it will open you up and allow for easier entry. But, do not think this position is only pleasurable for High Congress! Regardless of size, the Widely Open Position ensures that not much effort is exerted during sex, so that stamina for both people is increased. This is a very powerful position that can have sex last for as long as you would like it to, and neither person should find themselves getting tired quickly. It is also an intimate position, as the man gazes down upon the woman, and she gazes back up at him. Both people have their hands free if they so choose, so that they may caress each other's bodies. Men should make use of the fact that the woman's breasts are readily available to him, and he should play with them and stimulate them accordingly.

- The Yawning Position

The Yawning Position has the woman begin by lying flat on her back. From here, she will need to open up her thighs as wide as possible, and then raise them in the air until her thighs are against the bed, close to the sides of the body. To assist in keeping them open, she should grasp her thighs or ankles and hold them apart. The man will then lay or kneel in between her legs and can begin penetrating her.

- The Expanding Position

A slight variation from The Yawning Position also has the woman laying on her back with her legs widely spread apart. The difference that separates the two, however, is that the woman will not use her hands in order to assist her in keeping her legs apart. She may place her hands behind her head in a relaxed pose, or she may use her hands to caress the man's body. Whatever she chooses, she will need to keep her legs open naturally which can get tiring after some time. In order to offset the fatigue this position can cause, the woman can keep one leg sprawled out to the side but resting on the floor, while then raising the other leg up and away from her body. Here she will still be expanded open, but she can switch between which leg is on the ground in order to rest.

- The Position of Indrani

Closing out the three recommended positions for High Congress is The Position of Indrani, which is also known as the Position of the Wife of Indra. To get into this pose, the woman will lay on her back and spread her thighs open. She will bend so that her thighs are on the ground on either side of her. Her legs should fold on top of her thighs, with her claves resting on the back of each thigh. This is a very tricky position and requires a high degree of flexibility on the woman's part. If you are unable to master it on your first go, simply bend the thighs back towards the floor as much as possible, and then work towards it over time. Even in the Kama Sutra, it is noted that this is a position that requires much practice, so do not feel discouraged if it does not come naturally to you.

- The Side Clasping Position

The first of the Low Congress positions, the Side Clasping Position has both the man and woman laying on their side. To begin, the man should lay down on his left side, and the woman will lay on her right side so that she is facing him. Keeping her legs tightly pressed together, and him with his legs tightly together, he should then press himself against the woman's body and enter her from this position. Both the partner's legs should remain in a straight posture for the entire duration, and their bodies should stay tightly pressed against each other. There will be no space for the man to caress the woman's breasts, but he can run his hands along her back and buttocks.

- The Supine Clasping Position

The Supine Clasping Position is actually the main version of the Clasping pair and is a bit easier to engage in than The Side Clasping Position. Here, the woman will lay flat on back, with her legs straight out and pressed together. Think of yourself like a plank of wood, with your body in a perfectly straight alignment. Now, the man will lay on top of the woman, matching her position. His legs should also be straight and pressed together, resting on top of the woman's legs. His body should press down against hers, and he can place his hands on either side of her so that he can prevent her from having to bear all of his weight. The many must then enter the woman from this position, not spreading her legs at all, so that her yoni remains tightly squeezed shut.

- The Pressing Position

The Pressing Position is less of a position, and more of a move to engage in during The Clasping Position. While the Kama Sutra does list it as its own position, it requires that you are already engaged in sex in order to complete. For this, the couple must already be engaged in either variation of The Clasping Position, although The Supine Clasping Position works best. Once you are engaged actively in sex, the woman will then use her thighs to press down tightly against the man's erection. Living up to its name, she will begin pressing tightly against it, squeezing it so as to add more pressure and tightness for him.

Tantric Sex

Tantra is improving nutrition. "Our sexual energy is one of our most powerful energies for health creation," said Christiane Northrup, m. D., author "Women's bodies, women's wisdom." "In conscious use of sexual energy... we can tap into a true source of youth and vitality."

TYPES OF TANTRA

Although not all forms are well documented, the Tantra path and what it is today are important.

1.   Buddhist Tantra

Because of its highly secrecy and strict regulations, Buddhist Tantra is extremely complex to practice. The practice of tantra in Buddhism is essentially to achieve cleansing and a state of enlightenment. The repetition of dharanis (buddhistic chants and mantras-like statements), extended yoga techniques (see TrulKhor), regulation of breaths of Pranayama and the application of different mudras are hand positions.

Buddhist TantraVajrayana teaches four different types of Tantra-Sarma traditions. These are CharyaTantra–the external purification of the mind, KriyaTantra –focused on achieving internal quietness, Yoga Tantra–concentrating emphasis on the sense of absolute space in a calm state, and the most elegant yoga Tantra.

2.   Hindu Tantra

In addition, the ancient teachings of Hinduism from Puranas contain a great deal of information which is taken from the supernatural TantraShastra. This is a very hidden and powerful science that Indians have been practicing for centuries and claims to open up supernatural powers. It is a whole set of techniques and practices linked to the strength, awareness and depth of a person's consciousness.

During Hindu tantra worship, tantric mantras (repeating words to aid concentration) are used to solve problems. We are meant to produce immediate results by awakening the power that stimulates spiritual growth. Mantras are expected to have four layers, including the word and its meaning, a sense of mantra, a deep knowledge and an understanding of the mantra.

Tantra scriptures and texts generally mention the worship of a Hindu goddess, revered as Shakti, in Hindu culture. Shakti refers to a complex part of the universe with various complexities such as a seductive woman, celestial power, a devoted daughter, mother-nature and more. Shakti can manifest in different ways, and in any form, her divine power can be. She is also the ecstasy or divine tantric love and is often regarded as the "action."

There are three tantric practices of Indian tantra that all reflect Shiva's powers. These are, Vama–an impure tantra, Dakshina–a mixed existence for health, and Madhyama.

3.   Neo Tantra or New Age

The adoration of New Age and Neo Tantra has grown in popularity in the western world and reinterpreted Hindu and Buddhist traditions. This modern, contemporary activity is often called Neotantra. When time went on, some of the old outdated tantra teachings were re-opted for a modern lifestyle. These new teachings are still very closely related to the origins of Tantra and manly concentrate on the importance of sexuality and sensuality to reach a path to the God.

This practice now mixes tantric yoga and sexuality with a hidden spiritual energy for many Neotantricans. It has also developed into a tantric sex that storms the world and uses many physical and sexual aspects of tantra, while eliminating many religious practices. Once again, this is an example of the continuous integration of old tantra which adapts to a modern, new world and society.

4.   Yoga Tantra

An ancient cornerstone of knowledge is the already well-known history and dignity of yoga. Yoga uses very similar tantra techniques, such as breathing and body poses, in its entity. Yoga methodologies also concentrate particularly on awareness and connection so there's no surprise that yoga and tantra are directly linked.

The first cycle always becomes conscious of these wishes and sexual forces and then through movement interacts with your body to release them. This helps you not only to exhume sexual energy enjoyably, but also to balance your mind while finding peace.

These tantric texts were ambiguous and only intended to be understood by those who practiced the secret tantric arts closely.

The next time we see a significant emergence of Ancient Tantra is when it spread in India in the 11th and 12th centuries. The' Tantrikas' who were practitioners of tantric arts studied and taught it. They believed that those without the knowledge of tantra had a life unrelated and unbalanced to others.

What is Tantra History?

• Tantra dates back to 300 CE

• First in India by Hindu and Buddhist Scriptures

• Tantra then widespread throughout the Western world

• Tantrikas were masters who taught and studied Tantra

• Elements of Tantra can be found in the Buddhism, Hinduism & Yoga.

TANTRA AS A LIFESTYLE AND ITS BENEFITS

The ancient Sanskrit philologist Pādieini tells us that the tantra is related to the ideals of the holy mantras and offers spiritual freedom in medieval texts. He describes people who mastered tantra as "one who is self-dependent, one who is his own master, the most important thing for himself."

We know from this that tantra is not only designed to raise sexual consciousness, but also the awareness as a whole. Those who practice the tantra way of life use old tantra philosophies and merge them in a new manifestation of the tantra way of life. This can of course, involve sexual elements of tantra, such as sexual freedom, but this is not always the case.

Tantric practice not only helps deal with the positive aspects of your life, such as sexuality and well-being but also with the negative areas to be overcome. You can focus on areas such as your anxiety, emotional difficulties, and your confidence through tantric consciousness. Seeing things in tantric eyes helps you to discover an enlightened and enjoyable everyday life.

So, living a tantric lifestyle appears to be all about internally connecting in yourself and getting the ability to use your consciousness to improve your life.

What's a Tantric style of living?

- Tantric exercises can be used in order to focus on your life

- It's about liberation and self-knowledge

- You can resolve problems and fears challenging

- It can help with trust and understanding

- It does not have to include sexual elements but can if you want.

SEX AND TANTRA

Looking at Hindu tantra scriptures, the main focus seems to be on creating a universe. The balance of feminine and male power leads to a positive sexual outcome and to a connective sexual illumination. The concept of tantric teaching in Buddhist tantra is that sexual energy can be used to increase the awareness of all areas of your life.

The more intensive and pleasurable your relationship is with your partner, the greater the degree of sex and all areas of your life will improve. We use a variety of tantra resources to cultivate communication and concentrate the gain on sexual pleasure.

It is all good and good that these former Hindu and Buddhist philosophies include the sexual reference to their tantric teachings, but what exactly do people do when they indulge in tantric sex in the world of today? I hear you! I hear you! Let's further dive.

How does Tantra have to do with sex?

- Tantra scriptures identify the connection between sexual energy
- All about achieving connective sexual enlightenment
- Buddhist teachings suggest tantric sex brings a higher awareness
- There are different tantric sex practices
- New generation tantric sex workers can use it to lift their sex lives

TANTRIC SEX IN PRACTICE

Tantric sex is the most recent type of tantra. And as a result of its exciting nature, it has now become a media interest in the sexual corner. This incorporates many of the ancient Indian and Buddhist celestial relation lessons, but it also blends them with traditional sexual philosophies. Tantric gender can be regarded as a profound spiritual mode of lovemaking without the religious rituals of ancient tantra forms.

The practice of prolonged sex without ejaculation is one of the most popular tantric teachings derived from tantric meditation and awareness. The idea is to increase perception of anticipation by what some call sexual meditation.

If you stop and think, if we stop, slow down and take a breath, we can immediately be in the moment and absorb every sensation or emotion. Meditation can and does help many of us to overcome everyday obstacles. Why should we not use the same focus power to improve our ties, increase intimacy and achieve better orgasms most importantly?

What Are the Techniques of Tantric Sex?

- Tantric sex has many mental and physical methods
- ' Slowing Down' improves sensitivity and relation to your partner
- One well-known method is delayed ejaculation or long-lasting pleasure
- There are different tantric sex positions

•   Other tantric sex strategies include meditation and breathing practice

TANTRA AND TANTRIC MASSAGE

Now that we have comprehended what tantra is and the various ways people utilize it. Let's dive into the art of tantric massage. However, the overall objective of tantra and tantra massage is the same achieving a state of extreme happiness. This is provided by the tantric massage based on the influence of illuminated touch and using tannic prolonged ejaculation techniques.

Contrary to other forms of massage, tantra massage uses body to body to provide a godly sexual experience. The goal is to deliver waves of pleasure by taking the body to its climax and down again and again. If sexual energy is released, it is a strong and euphoric orgasm that replaces daily ejaculation.

What Is Tantric Massage?

•   It uses prolonged ejaculation strategies to give an amazing climax

•   Tantric massage is a sexual technique derived from tantras

•   The focus is usually on sensation and touch

•   Tantric masseuses use their entire bodies to massage you

•   Authentic elements can be present, depending on the masseuse

TANTRIC SEX BENEFITS

You can improve your sexual health naturally through tantric yoga and gender. Tantric Yoga provides many exercises that lead to a solid and blissful life, including a powerful combination of asana, mantra, mudra, bandha, and chakra. Tantric sex is a slow type of intimacy that can enhance closeness and a connection between the mind and the body that often results in intense orgasms. That combination, with a strong connection between body, mind, and spirit along with frequent, intense sexual orgasms, should enable loving couples to increase pineal and hypo-physical secretion.

- Tantric Sex Improves Sexual Health

Many say that tantric sex has a rejuvenating effect, enhancing the sexual health of men and women. Frequent orgasms can alter body chemistry, as one of the simulations of the brain wave. Depression and stress can go away. The sexual health of a woman can be greatly improved.

Tantric gender can be affected by endocrine glands for more HGH, dopamine, DHEA, and testosterone. Brain chemistry can be affected. Scientific and medical studies have shown that gender significantly improves health by enhancement of blood circulation, detoxification of body breathing and improving cardiovascular, endocrine /immune and nervous functions. For example, a study conducted by Wilkes University found that lovemaking produces an antibody called immunoglobulin A or IgA at least twice a week which can protect the body from disease.

- Orgasms Strengthening the Immune System

Orgasms can minimize anxiety and make you feel happier and happy. Others claim that it can also extend your life, boost your immune system and improve your overall health. To confirm these findings, however, more clinical studies are needed. Can semen sexual exposure combat depression and increase moods both in women and men? It can also be found that risky and unsafe sex can lead to depression while safe sex can provide mood, emotional connections, and intimacy, according to a Rebecca Burch report. Therefore, men and women may benefit significantly from increasing the sexual quantity and quality in a discreet, healthy and natural way through tantric sex. Tantric sex focuses on the advantages of expanding sexual activity to improve intimacy and health benefits.

Possible Benefits of Constant Orgasms, Women's Health, and Tantric Sex

Frequent orgasms can benefit the sexual health of a woman. There is this huge difference between a normal orgasm and a tantric orgasm. Ordinary orgasms last for a short period and remain isolated in sex organs. Theoretically, tantric sex orgasms involve the whole body, mind, and spirit and last for hours.

According to ancient traditions, to achieve the advantages of a tantric orgasm, the shakti or power, and the kundalini, each of the chakras must penetrate the upward spinal cord (energy vortexes in the subtle body). It must enter the central nervous system of the brain and the endocrine head office— the hypothalamus and the hypophysis that regulate changes in our sexual health.

Tantric sex devotees claim that normal, strong orgasms increase the hormone level of the orgasm, oxytocin. We also agree that the levels of oxytocin and your orgasms influence your mood, your enthusiasm, your social skills, and your emotions.

TANTRIC SEX POSITIONS

As we have discovered, tantric sex fundamentals involve concentrating on an advance play until you are ready to reach an explosive end rather than focusing on orgasm as your ultimate goal. Having tried some of the above moves, you could try moving to some tantra sex. The following tantric sex positions encourage you to practice tantric lovemaking with your partner and develop intimacy and make your two happy.

    1. Lotus Legs

Although this may be part of your daily love sessions, making this tantric sex position gradually rather than quickly brings a tantric twist into your routine. To do this, a woman must lie on the mattress, sitting on the edge of her butt. The male faces her and places her straight legs on her feet. This position allows the woman to float in bliss deep connection and comfort.

    2. Reverse Seated Hug

For some, the reverse seated embrace may be a challenge, but the reverse seated position offers the opportunity to be more relaxed. Sit down with your partner wrapping your arms around you in a kind of' backwards embrace' pose. Enjoy a slow rhythm in close sensual contact with the body.

3. Spooning

Even if spooning is already a common practice, you could add a switch in tantric sex that lifts this sex position to a new degree of ecstasy. Arrange yourself side by side and close in a spoon position. Hold one another and begin to breathe in a coordinated way. Use this time to encourage your hands to wonder and slowly turn towards penetration when you both exhales.

Sexual Fantasies

You probably have fantasies and fetishes you don't even know about.

They are lodged in there, in the deeper reaches of your subconscious, and simply haven't had a chance to expose them yet.

When I first started having sex, and for about a year and a half after, I had no clue I had a fantasy to dominate my partner. I didn't even know what that meant until it happened.

I didn't know that I would find it really hot to tie my partner up, and that my partner would find it really hot as well.

I didn't know that the thrill of getting caught while having sex in public would consume my thoughts for a period of time.

At this point in time, I don't have any strong role-playing fantasies. But I am completely open to them, even though my acting skills are crap.

And who knows, maybe I do have a powerful role-playing fantasy lodged in there somewhere. There's only one way to find out. I've got to try it.

So, how do fantasies arise out of our subconscious?

I have a theory that a lot of them come from the sexual ideas we were subject to when we were growing up.

I watched a lot of porn in my pubescent days, and as you watch more and more of it, you start going deeper and deeper into the rabbit hole. That may have had an impact on my sexual psyche, and I wouldn't be surprised if it's the same for many people.

If you grew up in a sexually closed-off environment, where you were shamed for expressing your sexuality, you may have been compelled to rebel against it, becoming more open-minded and experimental in the process. So, the experiences you had in your early sexual development may have had an impact on the fantasies and fetishes you have today.

If you can observe the fantasies you have today, try looking into your past and see if you can find their roots. It may help you understand why you have them, and in turn, help you understand your partner's fantasies and fetishes.

So, if fantasies reside in our subconscious, how do we unlock them?

I believe that the key to unlock these fantasies is made out of the trust you have in one another.

As this trust builds, your mind relaxes, opening the doors to many things (sexual and non-sexual) that allow themselves to be expressed.

It may come in the form of a desire being blurted out randomly in the middle of a sexual conversation. It may come out after a few drinks and your words are flowing out more comfortably than usual. It may come out in the middle of passionate sex, when one of you screams out exactly what they want to be done do them.

As you become more comfortable having sexual conversations, that feeling of weirdness starts to go away. Discussing where you want to eat dinner and discussing a new sex toy you want to try becoming just as natural to talk about.

For those in casual relationships, you start to initiate these conversations more frequently with people you're attracted to, naturally filtering out the people who aren't comfortable discussing it, and naturally filtering in the people who are comfortable. This leads to increased overall sexual compatibility and openness.

These sexual conversations lead you two into the deeper reaches of your desires.

Maybe there's a fantasy you've masturbated to a few times. You begin considering asking your partner if they want to try it. You are a little bit uncomfortable because it's only something you have fantasized about. You have never considered actually making it a reality.

But you and your partner have become so much more comfortable discussing this stuff that it doesn't seem nearly as strange as it would have a while back. So, you say, "What the hell, why not? Let's see where this thing takes us."

And so, you discuss it, you find out that your partner has fantasized about the exact same thing. Suddenly, you both get that feeling of nervous excitement in the pit of your belly telling you that you're about to have another pivotal experience.

As you share more sexual experiences, the connection grows further. Every experience becomes your little secret that only you two have intimate knowledge about.

This permeates your connection in many ways, through inside jokes as you walk down the street, through a quick glance when someone says something related to your experience together, and through the subtleties of your sexual flow in the bedroom.

All of these things can compound upon each other, leading to spontaneous expressions of these fantasies and fetishes in the bedroom. Without any sort of premeditation, you suddenly get a desire that you've never had before.

You are naturally submissive, but at this moment in time, all you want to do is dominate them.

You have never told your partner how you want to be touched before, but you've suddenly got this unrelenting urge to be touched a certain way, so you whisper it in their ear and make it happen.

These fantasies and fetishes act like little mysteries of the subconscious. Clues pop up all around until in one instant the solution reveals itself and the mystery is solved.

It's an interesting area of sexuality to navigate. There are tons of fantasies and fetishes to choose from (well, I guess in most cases, it's not really a choice). Just go to a porn site and look at the categories. Almost every one of them is a different fantasy or fetish.

I have provided a list of these fantasies and fetishes to show you what is available, and to possibly help you realize that the ones you hold, the ones you feel the most uncomfortable about, are actually quite normal to have.

I would assume that you are certainly not the only one in the world that has this fetish. But if you are, good for you! You can be a trendsetter. There is really no reason to be ashamed of these fantasies.

If you are with a person you trust and who trusts you back, if you have solid communication going on, and if you have become more and more comfortable discussing your sex life and have shared sexual experiences, you should be in a more than ideal environment to express these desires.

Here is a list of some of the more prominent sexual fantasies and fetishes I could find. Just going through this list might unlock something for you.

- Anal sex
- Anal play
- Bondage
- BDSM (Bondage and Sadomasochism)
- Pretending your strangers meeting each other and going home together
- Teacher and student
- Prisoner and prison guard
- Doctor and patient
- Nurse and patient
- Maid or house cleaner
- Having sex with a coworker
- Having sex with someone you have just met
- Having sex with someone older than you
- Having sex with someone younger than you (of legal age, of course)

- Having sex with multiple people at the same time
- Being completely submissive
- Being completely dominant
- Striptease
- MILFs
- Watching other people have sex
- Squirting
- Having sex on an airplane
- Orgies
- Voyeur (being watched while having sex)
- Different nationalities
- Sexy lingerie
- Gangbang
- Masturbation
- Being sexual with someone that wouldn't constitute a part of your chosen sexual orientation
- Using toys
- Filming each other
- Anilingus
- Footjobs and feet
- Dressing up in school uniforms
- Cheerleader fantasy
- Playing cop and criminal
- Hooking up with the delivery person
- Having sex in public
- Being spanked

- Thrusting into your partner's mouth

- Golden shower (peeing)

- Gagging

- Femdom (feminine domination)

- Fisting

- Deepthroating

- Talking dirty

Odds are, reading some of those may have made you feel uncomfortable. That's alright, especially if you haven't heard of them before.

Don't be judgmental, of yourself or others. It's next to impossible to control what we desire. If your partner expresses something to you that you don't feel comfortable with, react tactfully. If you don't, you could hurt them and tarnish all of the trust you have built together.

Talking About Sexual Fantasies and Fetishes

You can sit down with your partner, write down all of the fantasies you have and would like to try, then trade papers and compare. It's usually much easier to start out communicating this way than to jump straight into a conversation about it.

But if you're comfortable enough, by all means, don't shy away from having that conversation.

Building Your Carnal Confidence

Talking is supposed to be easy. After all, you've been doing it since you were a kid. But why on earth is dirty talking so darn hard? The truth is that even the most talkative individuals and even the most imaginative writers find playful pillow talk a bit challenging. Some words may seem erotic on print but might sound downright embarrassing when spoken out loud. Even the most sexually confident men and women will eventually come across a naughty word that would make them blush from head to toe. That's because traditionally, sex has always been about the deed.

At first, dirty talking would make you feel like you're somehow stripping your clothes off over and over again. With every word, it's like a new layer comes off and you'll wait anxiously as to how your partner will react. Will he like it? Will she get turned off?

So, how do you make sure that all that sexy talking won't send your lover packing?

First, practice with yourself.

Your vulgar vocab may initially shock you but who cares? You're the only one who'll be able to hear it anyway. Begin by masturbating. Then, start talking dirty to yourself. At this point, you don't have to have a rich vocabulary. Just use simple words. Focus on the pleasure and think out loud. Blurting out an honest sentence like: "Oh yeah, that feels good." is already a hundred times hotter than staying silent.

Next, imagine that you're having sex with your lover. It's what you do when you masturbate, anyway. If you're a guy, as you slip your cock into your lubed-up fist, imagine that it's her pussy. And so instead of saying: "Oh yeah, that feels good.", say: "Oh yeah, your pussy feels good."

If you're a woman, imagine his cock as you slide your fingers in and out of you. And so instead of saying: "Oh yeah, that feels good.", say: "Oh yeah, your cock feels so good."

Still, words like "good" are way too broad. When it comes to sexy talk, the more specific you are, the greater the impact. As you continue imagining that you're making love to your partner, describe the feelings in your head. Bring life to those sensations with adjectives.

Examples:

"Oh yeah, your pussy is so fucking tight!"

"Oh yeah, your cock is so fucking thick!"

But then again, anyone's cock can be thick. Anyone's pussy can be tight. For dirty talk to be powerful, it must hit home. Moreover, when using adjectives, you must be careful and make sure you stick to the truth as much as possible. For instance, don't describe a man's cock as "thick" when you both know that it isn't.

The next step, therefore, is to consider your partner. What's he/she like? What do you think he/she would like to hear most? What do you think he/she needs to hear most?

Is he's constantly worried about his size? Say something like: "Baby, I love how your cock fits me perfectly."

Is she self-conscious about her heavy boobs? Tell her how burying your face in them feels like heaven.

See, you're getting good at this already! As you get more comfortable and more talkative, masturbate and practice your dirty talk with a tape recorder. Listen to yourself. This way, you'll know whether you need to talk more or to talk less, to speak louder or softer, or whether you need to take the naughtiness up or down a notch.

Form a positive attitude and an open mind.

The source of most people's hang-ups is the idea that dirty talk somehow cheapens them, their partners, or their relationships. To become erotically eloquent, you need to get over the myth that dirty words make the act of sex unclean. One thing you need to understand is that a person's sexual persona is just one aspect of himself/herself. Who your lover is in the sack does not make up all of him/her? It is not who he/she is outside the bedroom. Your genitals are not dirty. Your partner's genitals are not dirty. By using straightforward words to refer to them (ex: cunt, penis, pussy, cock, breasts, boobs, vagina, balls, etc.), you are asserting the fact that these body parts are not to be ashamed of but instead deserve to be appreciated and therefore, mentioned.

Try this activity:

Stand naked in front of a mirror. Look at your genitals and touch them. Observe them. Determine and describe what you like most about them.

Ex:

My breasts are a nice handful. My nipples are small and pretty. I love how sensitive they are!

or

My breasts are big and generous. They're soft and bouncy and I love playing with them!

Make sure that you concentrate on the positive things. And never, ever compare yourself with the airbrushed vaginas and surgically enhanced penises in porno films and magazines. Ex: If you're conscious about how your labia minora is an outie, think about how awesome it is that your guy gets to have some flesh to nibble on during cunnilingus.

Talk to your lover about sex. It's the healthy thing to do.

The more comfortable you are with discussing sex with your lover, the easier it is for you to transition to dirty talking. After having sex, move close to your partner and confess to him/her how you felt. Mention the bedroom tricks and lovemaking positions that you liked the most. Tell your lover which things you want her/him to do again and again.

Ex: I went crazy when you put a vibrator on my clit while you went down on me. I can't wait for you to do it again.

Be specific. Get graphic. Sure, it was hot when your lover did it to you but hearing the act narrated through your lips will make it even hotter. Observe your lover's reaction. His/her response will help you gauge how he/she feels about smutty speech.

Never judge.

The bed should be a judgment-free zone. Just as you don't criticize your partner when he/she shows you his/her body, refrain from criticizing your lover when he/she bares his/her thoughts. Understand that to speak openly entails trust. To be vocal before, during, or after intercourse makes one more vulnerable. Therefore, during sexy talk, stifle the urge to laugh or to react indignantly. Don't rebuke your lover for his/her poor choice of words during sex or foreplay. Talk about it at least a few hours later.

Ex: You know when we were making love and you called me a cum dumpster? Well, that was a little too dirty for me."

Dirty talk is not a license to be disrespectful.

To stop dirty talk from being a tad too dirty for your tastes, create a set of rules with your partner. Talk about which words you're okay and not okay with.

Example: "I'm fine with being called a gutter whore. Just don't call me a bang hole."

Great lovemaking is all about giving and take. It's easy enough for the more talkative partner to dominate the dirty dialogue. That said, view dirty talking as an opportunity to allow the more silent person to verbalize more. It's one way to get to know your lover in a deeper sense. Don't forget to take turns and to always be on the same page when acting out roles. If one is the slave, then the other must be the master. There can't be two masters at one time. Moreover, being able to put yourself in the shoes of the listener and the talker will enable you to form a sensible perspective.

"Hey honey, let's dance the chocolate cha cha."

Does this colloquial term for anal sex conjure images of feces? If it does, then you don't have to use it in your coital conversations. Feel free to make your own lust lingo that you'll feel comfortable with. Remember, the objective of dirty talk is to arouse you and not to gross you out. More than, making your own secret dirty dialect will serve to deepen the intimacy that you share with your lover.

Roleplay

Just like you can't drive a car without warming up the engine first, you shouldn't engage in sexual intimacy without warming up the body via foreplay. When we think of foreplay the first thing that comes to mind is the physical aspect of it, but there is much more to the act than just touching. Here, we are going to dive into what exactly foreplay is, some tips and tricks on making foreplay better, why foreplay is so important, and how you can incorporate foreplay into your everyday life.

So, what is foreplay?

Foreplay is anything leading up to sex that arouses you and your partner. It can be physical, mental, or verbal and it can begin moments before sex or days before. This is where consent begins, as you both acknowledge that you are interested in having sex with one another. From there you tease and play, turning each other on and getting your minds and body ready.

As we mentioned, there are many different types of foreplay, but the four most common are physical, mental, visual, and verbal. Many of these are intertwined and connected, but it is important to talk about each separately so as to really pick out some great tips and advice. Let us dive in and look at each of the four more closely!

Physical Foreplay

Physical foreplay is the one most people think of when talking about this subject. It's easy to picture what physical foreplay looks like and what it involves. Typically utilized right before having sex, physical foreplay is anything that involves touching yourself or the other person. It can be via massage, mutual masturbation, slow caresses, or anything else that you enjoy.

Our bodies respond powerfully to physical touch, so this is a very important part of the sex process. Without physically stimulating our partner, they may not be ready to engage in sexual intercourse. For women, you want to be wet and ready for penetration, whereas men need to be hard and erect. In order to get to these places, you can physically arouse your partner by trying some of the following:

- Mutual Masturbation – By engaging in mutual masturbation you can achieve multiple goals that will enhance sex. Firstly, you are manually arousing your partner and stimulating their genitals in a way that prepares them for intercourse. Additionally, you can use this as an opportunity to show your partner how you like to be touched. You know your body best, so show them the speed, pressure, and areas that really get you going.

- Sensual Massage – Break out those oils and go to town on your partner's body! Not only will the soft touches arouse your partner physically, but there is nothing more relaxing than receiving a massage. The more relaxed your body is and the more comfortable you feel, the more likely you are to let go and really enjoy sex. Try taking turns so that you both are able to reap the benefits of this sexy foreplay.

- Kiss More Than Their Lips – Instead of using your hands to trace the curves of their body, why not use your mouth? Spend time getting to know every inch of them by kissing them slowly from their head to their toes. Find the areas that make them shiver and the run your tongue slowly across those secret spots. You may be surprised at what non-sexual areas actually create a sexual response. The neck, earlobes, nipples, and thighs are all great places to explore, but beyond that you can try their ribs, stomach, behind the knees, and anywhere else you dare to go.

- The Joy of Oral – Oral sex can be both foreplay as well as sex by itself, it simply depends on what you and your partner like. If using it as foreplay, however, this is a very obvious way to get that party started. Going down on your partner is sure to arouse them and make them ready for what's to come.

- Take Control – Some people like things to be slow and intimate, some people like it hard and rough, and others enjoy a mix of the two. If you're on the rougher and tumble side of things, then foreplay can be a great place to let out that animalistic side of you. So long as everything is safe and consensual, go ahead and let lose by grabbing your partner and pinning their hands above their head. Biting and choking can be extremely arousing for some people, and if you and your partner are into this then go ahead and play! Taking control of the situation can be an incredibly powerful way of showing your partner how badly you want them and can make them feel sexy and desired. Plus, being overpowered allows you to let loose a bit more freely, so be a freak and get naughty!

- Don't forget the basics – While sexy massages and being handcuffed to a bed are all great ways to play around before sex, it's important that you don't forget to engage in the very basics that work wonders. Kissing is such a powerful tool that many people overlook because it seems so simple and common. But a great make-out session can work just as well, or even better, than any of the above tips. That also goes for actions like running your fingers up and down their sides or spooning in bed. Foreplay doesn't have to be crazy or excessive, it just needs to work.

Mental Foreplay

Mental foreplay is anything that engages the mind and make us think or visualize something erotic and sexy. Unlike physical foreplay which is typically in the moments leading up to sex, mental foreplay can begin hours, or even days in advance. Think back to before you ever had sex with your partner for the first time. Maybe you waited a few days, weeks, or months before you finally got to have sex with them. In that time though you probably thought a lot about sex and what it would be like when you had it. You mentally pictured your partner naked or engaging in sexual acts with you. More than likely these thoughts got your quite aroused, and when the moment finally happened you were more than ready to go.

That's just one example of what mental foreplay can involve, and when it comes to gender differences, mental foreplay is often more successful with women than it is with men. While both genders equally love physical foreplay, women, on average, tend to become more aroused by thoughts and fantasies that play out on their minds. Are you really looking to turn a woman on? Try some of these mental foreplay tips:

- Delay Sex - Just like when you first started dating, the thought of having sex with someone can be a powerful turn-on. Bring back that old spark by holding off on sex for a few days, or even a week, and really get your partner thinking about how badly they want it. Sex every day can be amazing, but when you break up that routine you can throw your partner off and get inside their head. One thing that's important to note here, however, is that you should communicate your game plan with your partner. If you suddenly start rejecting them and ignoring their advances it can end up creating hurt feeling and even confidence issues. You're trying to turn them on, not permanently turn them off, so tell them you are going to make them wait until the beg you for it! Knowing they can't have something will make them want it even more and guaranteed they will be thinking about having sex with you non-stop.

- What's Your Fantasy? – Set the scene ahead of time by letting your partner know what your ultimate fantasy is. Maybe you want to be surprised in the kitchen while making dinner? Or maybe you love the idea of playing teacher and student? It doesn't matter what your fantasy is, or even if it's possible, it just matters that you share it in as much detail as possible. Paint a mental picture for your partner and you break down exactly what would happen in your fantasy. Tell them what you would be wearing, how you would be touched, and exactly how that sex would be. If you're feeling extra creative, why not write your partner an erotic short story? Give it to them and let them read it in private, or even read it out loud to them! However, you want to share, go ahead and open up. And who knows, maybe that story will lead to your fantasy coming true.

- All Day Foreplay – One of the absolute best ways to really get your partner turned on is to utilize all day foreplay. Start by sending your partner a saucy text message in the morning, and follow it up throughout the day with sexy texts about what you like, what you're feeling, and what you want to do when they get home. Maybe you throw in a sexy snapshot, or some suggestive emojis. However, you like to do it, playing with your partner all day long is sure to build up that sexual tension. It can be even more arousing because it is in a space that is not reserved for sex, like at work. When you're in a different environment it can be shocking and more erotic as you feel like you're secretly being naughty. Not only does it get their mind going, but it also shows that you can't stop thinking of them and there is nothing sexier than being desired.

- Clean the House - Aright, so this may sound like the least sexy thing of all but taking on chores and getting things done can be incredibly sexy. Mental foreplay isn't just about making someone think about sex, it's also about making them not think at all. When your partner comes home, they don't want to think about dinner and household chores, because if they are then they certainly won't be thinking about sex. Ease their mind and relax them by ordering in some food and taking care of the chores. When they walk through that door and see a clean house and no work for them, they are a million times more likely to want to jump on you. Also, it's a simple way to show your partner that you care, and that in itself can be a huge turn on. Taking on chores that aren't yours, or just putting in a bit of extra effort can go a very long way.

Visual Foreplay

Just like mental foreplay, which was more geared towards women, men have a favorite type of foreplay as well: visual foreplay. Women's arousal begins with their minds, but men are turned on by what they see in front of them. Visual foreplay can lead to mental foreplay, and the two are often connected, but it deserves its own category because there is the added bonus of being able to actually see without being able to touch.

From sexy pictures to erotic dances, visual foreplay can be fun and arousing. Just think, why do so many men enjoy going to strip clubs? There is no option to actually engage in any sexual activity, but the environment itself is charged with sexual tension and desire. Being able to look and not touch can make you want it even more, so try these visual tricks to really get your partner turned on:

- Send a Sexy Snap – If you are in a relationship that has a significant amount of trust then you can try sending your partner sexy photos of yourself. These do not have to be fully nude pictures, but anything seductive will work. Maybe you are wearing a lower cut blouse, or a short skirt. How about simply biting your lip and sending that? Sexy pictures can involve anything, from being fully clothed to completely naked, it's whatever you are comfortable sharing. The visual of seeing you naked is sure to turn

- Give a Lap Dance – Who needs to spend money at the strip club when you can turn your own bedroom into a private one? Whether you're a professional dancer or you have two left feet, a lap dance is sure to be appreciated by your partner. Let them watch your body move as you tease them, never letting them quite touch. The visual of you in a sexy outfit, dancing just for their eyes, will turn them on like you've never seen before.

- Watch Porn Together – Even though most people don't like to admit it publically, the majority of us watch pornography. Watching it alone is always enjoyable but watching it with a partner can be just as fun. It may feel awkward at first, but find something you both enjoy and dive in. Not only will it get you aroused, but maybe you both can pick out some tricks or positions that you want to try together. Remember, porn isn't real, and the people are actors, so don't feel bad if you can't perfectly recreate the acts you see. Just have fun and experiment, since that is what great sex is all about!

4. Verbal Foreplay

Unlike the other types of foreplay mentioned, verbal foreplay is more likely than the rest to be incorporated with other aspects and activities. Under mental foreplay we mentioned "all day play", and that includes a lot of verbal aspects, such as texting and talking. Sharing a fantasy with a partner creates a mental image, but it also requires you speaking and communicating in order to make that happen.

Without great communication you more than likely won't even get close to having sex, because you need to have both a talk and consent before you begin. From telling a partner you find them sexy to spilling every last detail of your greatest fantasy, verbal foreplay is the most important aspect to having sex happen. Let's break down some ways in which we can take verbal foreplay even further:

- Talk Dirty to Me – People tend to be quite divided over dirty talk, with some people absolutely loving it and others refusing to ever partake in the act. While dirty talk is extremely effective, it also tends to be a bit embarrassing and it can make someone feel a bit unsure and self-conscious. If you're wanting to give a try but you aren't confident, start slow and simple. Dirty talk doesn't need to be aggressive or outrageous, and instead you can begin by simply saying when something feels good. Tell your partner what you like, ask them to touch you in a certain way or in a specific place. This is all part of talking dirty. The more you try it out, the more your confidence will grow until you are ready to start getting more detailed.

- Have Phone Sex – If you've ever been in a long-distance relationship then you know the trials and tribulations that come with being away from your lover. Luckily with the internet we have the ability to see someone no matter where they live, but that doesn't mean we should discount the decades that people resorted to good old-fashioned phone sex. Even if you're not in a long-distance relationship, this is a great way to get someone's heart racing without even touching them. You could call your spouse while they are on their lunch break or go out for a walk and give them a ring. If you don't live with your partner this is even easier to accomplish, and instead of getting together you can simply have phone sex to get each other aroused. This is a great example as well of how foreplay doesn't always have to lead to actual sex, a concept we will get into more detail about below.

Most people think of foreplay as the build-up to sex, but it's important to remember that foreplay can be more than enough just on its own. If you only think of it as the appetizer, you miss out on how much fun it can be as a main course. Foreplay can be both intimate and extremely sexual and can easily lead to orgasms for both partners. Sometimes we aren't always in the mood for full on sex, but a little foreplay is just right.

During their period, some women aren't always up for vaginal intercourse, but that doesn't mean they aren't aroused and wanting to be touched. Foreplay is great for releasing some sexual tension and being intimate with your partner, in a way that is different from the norm.

With foreplay it is all about experimentation and trying something new. It's a perfect arena for practicing your communication skills, as this is where you want to be extremely vocal about your likes and dislikes. Tell your partner what feels good, moan, make noises, whisper your dark secrets, and touch every inch of them.

Dirty Talk

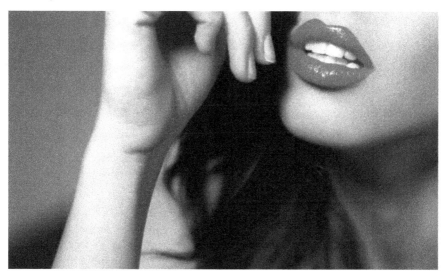

Talking dirty is another element that can truly enhance your relationship. And not only provides stimulation but it helps to improve communication. Regardless of if you are in a new relationship or a long-term one dirty talk is important. There are a variety of different reasons that this type of communication is important.

You already know how important communication is not only to the relationships you hold outside of the bedrooms, but also the ones that are more intimate. It makes sense that if communication is key prior to participating in a sexual encounter that it would also be important during the sexual encounter. It is appropriate to use dirty talk at any point in this type of experience. It can be used during foreplay or during the actual act of sex.

Some people think that talking dirty is intimidating but it really doesn't need to be. Being comfortable with your partner is going to make it exceptionally easy. Most people will admit that they enjoy a bit of dirty talk while in the throes of passion. It is quite uncommon for somebody to be completely against talking dirty while participating in sexual activities.

When people talk dirty in the bedroom it helps them to understand what they're comfortable with. If you are inexperienced in talking dirty it can be a bit tricky. This is especially true if you have a hard time with communication or there are simply words that are you are uncomfortable saying. Keep in mind that there are a variety of different terms for all of the words that you may find uncomfortable when trying to say them.

There needs to be some understanding that certain words outside of the bedroom may be completely unacceptable while they really turn you on while in the throes of passion. This is completely normal. It all comes down to communication. Perhaps you do not like the word pussy on a day to day basis but when your partner says it during times of sexual activity it really turns you on. This is fine as long as they have an understanding of when it is appropriate to use.

Using dirty talk is a great way to get your partner in the mood. When used during foreplay it can make the desire that your partner holds much higher. The enhancement of sexual pleasure can be noticed when the dirty talk is involved. Don't be afraid to get creative and use words or phrases that would not commonly occur in your day-to-day life.

Some people find that talking dirty is as important as foreplay. In fact, they really do go hand in hand. If you're trying to get your man or woman in the mood starting by whispering some dirty thoughts into their ear is almost always going to work. It provides them with the knowledge that you're interested in getting busy and can even help to encourage their sexual juices to get flowing.

It is commonly stated that people believe their sexual encounters are enhanced when the dirty talk is involved. It can be a bit surprising to your partner, but it is also, usually, very welcomed. Don't be afraid to add some dirty language when you guys are in the throes of passion. It really is a fun way to spice things up and take a step closer to your more adventurous side.

RULES

___

To ensure that you and your partner have a good time and experience using dirty talk, there definitely has to be some ground rules set prior to the activity itself.

This includes things to say and what not to say - not everyone would be turned on by, "mmm, your skin feels like my little baby brother's butt". For some, it could be borderline disturbing so it's crucial that these next few parts aren't skipped out.

- Find out what you and your partner like

A good rule of thumb is to have a mature, open and honest conversation about what you and your partner want to say or do before doing it. Even as you're doing it, it's good to have ongoing feedback about what you like or don't like, which is the best way to learn about each other. In other words, say what you want before sex – and say what you like during sex.

It may be difficult to talk about it without actually trying it out first, so experiment with each other to find out what you like or don't like. An easy way to find out is by asking, for example "Tell me all the places you want me to touch you…". Your partner will probably use the words he / she finds most erotic, helping you build up your bedroom vocabulary. Similarly, you can tell your partner what you want him/her to do to you.

If he or she is only interested in jumping you without engaging in conversation, then I'd suggest you really encourage your partner to open up or reconsider your relationship. Even fuck buddies can have a good conversation before getting into it – why do you think their sex is always so good?

- Choose your words

It'll also be good to find out if you and your partner prefer dirty talk to be sweet or risque; whether foul words turn you on or off; whether roleplay is on the table; what each other's fantasies are; what trigger words turn you on or off; or whether you like it loud or soft.

Setting up a preliminary list of words (say, top 10) to use or not use would be a good way to get started. This way, you'll both be on the same page and not be surprised by what is actually said by the other party. It also comes down to how comfortable you feel with your partner – the words you use shouldn't be weird or too vulgar; you should know your partner best from the open and honest conversation you would've had from before. For example, "You like that don't you, you are fucking whore?". Some (Most, I believe) would be offended and take that as derogatory, but there may be a select few out there who find it a huge turn on.

Talking about all these in advance does not make it less sexy; it's just being mature and respectful of your partner's needs and emotions. Because of that, it makes dirty talking even sexier.

- Establish ground rules

Besides coming up with a list of words to say, there are subtle accompanying actions that could make the sexual occasion more thrilling or completely awkward. One of the reasons some may feel uncomfortable talking dirty is the fear of sounding ridiculous or being rejected by a partner. Therefore, it's important to set some ground rules when you and your partner talk dirty to each other. Basic rules such as not laughing at each other (laughing together is fine) and not being judgemental are important as this affects overall self-esteem. It's essential to be respectful of each other.

It may be difficult to control the brain in the heat of the moment but making a conscious effort to think before you speak so as not to accidentally offend your partner is a priority. As a general rule, try not to highlight each other's size or insecurities. If your partner is insecure about the size of certain body parts, focus on how those parts feel instead. For example, say "Your erection is so hard" or "Your boobs are so soft". This switches the attention to how good they feel rather than on their size. With time, this will become second nature and even if you're in a polygamous relationship - this attention to detail will go a long way.

- Be genuine

Good dirty talk should come from the heart and ironically, should not follow a specific script. This book is meant to guide you with examples and dialogue but at the end of the day, you have to be your own person and use your own voice.

The first step would be to forget everything you've learned or heard in the movies or in porn. While some may be okay with it, the conversations could either come out really tacky or crude. Be yourself and say what comes to mind. Of course, a little practice will help in building up your confidence and comfort in dirty talking if you're not used to it.

You also don't need to have a deep husky voice or a sweet tone to talk dirty. It could be soft whispers, high pitched squeals, or low rhythmic grunts. Your dirty talk voice should come naturally from you and reflect the way you talk in your daily life or express a different side of your personality that you rarely get to explore. You could even have a few different dirty talk voices depending on the situation, mood, or roles that you're playing.

All these can add an element of surprise in your sexual routine, helping to heat things up in the bedroom even more. Experiment with different speeds of talking. Change the volume of your voice to suit different moods - try whispering when you want to be seductive and screaming when you're experiencing intense pleasure. Try it on your partner to see how he/she responds - you might find out something new about your partner that they even didn't know they liked before!

- Build Your Vocabulary

Let's face it - it's not easy to come up with fresh phrases or words to use (hence why you're reading this book), especially if you're new to dirty talking. The truth is, though, there are no strict guidelines or rules when it comes to dirty talk - it all depends on your desires and imagination. Of course, dirty talk can get pretty boring if you keep using the same phrases and words.

As such, it's good to expand your arsenal of dirty words through other mediums where possible - just preferably not from porn. The main reason why pornography should be the last resort is due to its lack of filter. Nobody watches porn because they want to be romantic. Yes, it's true that one of the most common forms of dirty talk involve foul words, but there's so much more to dirty talk than that.

Other than the examples provided, you can also read some raunchy erotica, watch some erotic and romantic films, and even learn to say some naughty things in a different language (some say that French is one of the sexiest languages in the world, but you can choose any language you want). If you or your partner have a favourite movie, poem, or song, you could even slip in some raunchy lines from those media into your dirty talk routine - I'm sure it will surprise and even delight them!

GETTING PAST THE AWKWARD PHASE OF TALKING DIRTY

No doubt about it, this is the hardest phase for you to get past when it comes to talking dirty, but you have to get past it. Hey, I get it. It can be a little awkward the first time. Not going to lie. All kinds of thoughts may go through your head. "Is he going to think I'm stupid? Is he going to think I'm a whore? Is he going to like it? This is supposed to feel good, but it just feels…. AWKWARD."

It's important to remember that most guys love it when you talk dirty. Why? Because half the time they're secretly wondering if you really want them the way that they want you to. Want to know something else? When you bring out your naughty side, you will have him aching for more because he knows you're going over to the forbidden side just for him. And he loves the fact that he's the one that has taken you there.

Keep in mind that there is nothing wrong with voicing your sexual desires and thoughts. Dirty talk is not dirty. It's only natural, and even if it isn't coming naturally to you, it will over time. Free your voice and allow yourself to rile him up like you've always wanted to.

Want me to let you in on a secret? If you can grasp what I'm about to tell you next and embrace it thoroughly, you can probably just skip the rest of the book and go straight to the examples. Seriously.

Enjoy the sex! Clear your mind of everything but satisfying your primal sexual urge. Feel it. Really feel it. Don't worry about what you look like, don't worry about what he's thinking. Just let the natural lust completely take over your mind and body.

Now, let your body tell your mind what to say. Tell him what you really want, when you want it. And just let go! Give in. Surrender completely to the passion. Once you're in this sexy state of mind, you are in control my dear. You will be playing on a different field and not give a damn about what anybody thinks. Your lust will be undeniable, and he will know it with every fiber in his body, especially the ones that count. Trust me. THIS is what he really wants anyway. The words will flow out of your mouth and naturally sound like a sexual soundtrack playing over and over in his head. Awkwardness… GONE. Congratulations, you just stepped over to the naughty side and you won't ever want to go back to silent, boring sex.

Got it? Good. Head on over and get started looking at your examples so you'll have the words to say when your body starts talking ;)

Hmmmm… are you thinking "Easier said than done?" Does the idea of talking dirty to your man still seem scary? That's perfectly normal. Hang in there with me and let's talk a little more to see if you can get comfortable with the idea before you nosedive right in. And don't worry.

Let Go of Fear:

Fear is actually what is holding most people back from talking dirty like they want to. In the bedroom there has to have been a time where you've wanted to tell him exactly what to do to drive you over that cliff, and when you talk dirty you can do just that. Something held you back, but there doesn't have to be that barrier anymore. Men don't even want that barrier to be there. Not at all! Women put it up, and women have to take it down.

It's common to have a fear of letting yourself speak freely, and this is both related to your sexuality and other things. You have to ask yourself why you're afraid to speak your mind and talk in that manner.

- Do you feel like he'll just laugh at you?

- Do you feel ashamed of your sexuality?

- Are you just not confident enough?

These are the three main reasons that people will stop themselves before they've even begun, setting themselves up for failure. If you want to reach the sexual heights that dirty talking can provide for the both of you, then you're going to need to bring out that bad girl warrior inside of you, be strong and fight through it!

You may be afraid of being sexual. Slut shaming is far too common, but enjoying your sexuality is a good thing. It's only natural to enjoy having sex, and we were programmed to do just that. Never feel ashamed of your sexuality! Instead, take charge of it, and that is what talking dirty can help you to do. Embracing your sexuality in the bedroom will be a game changer for you. You need to own it like the sex goddess you are.

If you're lacking confidence, the best thing to do is just to push past the fear that's holding you back. I don't know of anyone that was totally confident the first time they talked dirty. Talking dirty is what gives you more confidence. Nobody waits till they are confident they can run 10 miles before they start walking, right? Be kind of silly. Got to start somewhere and work up. Same here, naughty girl. You can't wait until you're totally confident to start talking dirty. Take that plunge and talk dirty to your man.

Sex Toys

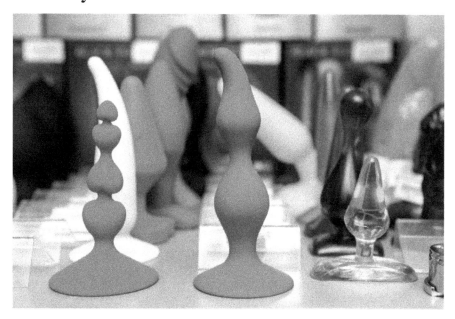

Vibrators and sex toys

Aside from a penis, a tongue, or fingers, a vibrator can be a woman's best friend. If you're a woman that doesn't have a vibrator (you poor, deprived thing!), you might want to consider getting one. Not only is it a great masturbation tool and a fine stress reliever, but it's also a wonderful way to share a sexual experience with your partner. Vibrators come in a variety of different shapes, sizes, styles, etc. You can get the old school, white plastic model, or you can go for the ultra-realistic looking dildo in the shape and size of your favorite male porn star.

How to get the best out of it

Some people view sex toys as something that is for those who have wild kinks or those who cannot perform without assistance of some sort. In reality, though, sex toys are designed to increase and enhance pleasure for anyone. By using sex toys, you do not have to engage in anything wild or anything that you are uncomfortable with. You are also not admitting that you have a sexual problem by using a sex toy.

One of the ways in which sex toys can improve your sex life is that they allow you to focus on one area of the body while the sex toy takes care of pleasure in another. For example, a sex toy that is designed to pleasure a woman's clitoris will do so while you can focus on her nipples or her vagina.

Finding the right toy

In order to choose the right sex toy for yourself, there are a couple of questions that you would need to answer first.

·   Is this toy to be used alone during masturbation?

·   Is it to be used with a partner?

·   Is it to be used with multiple partners?

·   Is it to be used for all of the above or two of the above?

·   Do you want it to have a vibrating function?

·   An insertion functions.

·   Will you use it anally?

·   Vaginally?

·   Both?

·   Do you want it to be customizable (depending on your mood or the partner you are with)?

Once you establish this, you will be able to narrow down your search. Answering all of these questions will help you to determine which type of sex toy is right for you (and your partner).

Sex position and sex toys

Once you've got your first four sex toys ready, it's time to combine this with some sex positions and begin exploring just how much pleasure the introduction of something new can bring. Of course, you can start getting a little more adventurous later once both partners are comfortable with the idea of using these toys in the bedroom. Until then, these positions will serve as a good first step to test the waters:

- The Missionary with Vibrator

Time to get back to basics once more as you slowly familiarize each other with the use of these sex toys. The woman will be lying down on her back on the bed, relaxed and ready. The man starts off slow and gentle, locating her clitoris with his fingers. Turn the vibrator on a low buzz, slowly bring it between her legs and place it so that it lightly touches her clitoris. The man then watches her facial expressions change as he tries varying amounts of pressure and speed settings of the vibrator. Occasionally take her by surprise by slipping a finger inside her vagina and find her G-spot while the vibrator is still going. Listen to her moans of desire for your cues to help her reach intense levels of pleasure. Adjust the speed when you're ready, increasing the speed as the woman gets wetter and wetter.

- Doggy Style with The Strap-On

The Doggy position, when combined with a strap-on creates a mecca of pleasure. This time, however, it is the man who is going to be in the Doggy position while the woman wears the strap on and do what you normally would do in this position. Be careful when playing with the man's anus, and don't forget to use lots of lube for this one.

- Seated Sex Position with the Vibrating Cock Ring

With the Cock Ring positioned at the base of the man's penis, vibrating and ready, the man sits in a chair while the woman sits on his lap, facing him with her legs around his waist and behind you. Have her stand up slightly, so she is hovering before she lowers herself onto the vibrating penis. Work together to move her body up and down on your penis. She can rotate her hips slightly backward, and the vibrating ring should stimulate her clitoris. The vibration of the ring will give her intense pleasure, and this position is ideal for a great male orgasm and a great female orgasm too.

Sex toys are devices or object a person may use to cause sexual stimulation. The tools are made to replace the pleasure that human genitalia would provide. Although there are vibrating toys, other forms of toys may provide pleasure without having to vibrate. These toys are readily available in sex shops and are available in a variety of types and purposes. It would be advisable for you to incorporate sext toys if only your partner advocates for it. You could use them before, during, and after sexual intercourse to initiate, maintain, and prolong sexual stimulation.

Types of Sex Toys

- Electro stimulators- These toys are available for both men and women and use electricity for stimulation. They work when placed on nerve endings, where they send signals to the brain. As a result, the brain releases pleasure hormones which then may lead to orgasm.

- Penetrative Toys- These are sex toys that are meant to make a penetration for sexual pleasure. They include a dildo which is a vibrating object used to penetrate either the anus or the vagina. Although there are different shapes of dildos, most resembles the shape of the penis. The most common types of dildos include strap-on and double penetration. Similarly, a horseshoe toy penetrates both the vagina and the anus at the same time to provide maximum stimulation and pleasure. A sex machine combines penetration with a rotational movement while a kegel exerciser improves the muscle tone of the vagina. There are love balls commonly inserted and lodged in the vagina for prolonged stimulation and eventually orgasm. Anal beads work similarly with the butt plugs, which are also embedded in the anus and make a smooth rotation to cause stimulation. Men like a massage on the prostate and enhance orgasm. Glass sex toys are made of clear glass and may sometimes aid in medical purposes. The glasses act as perfect temperature regulators as they penetrate in the anus or the vagina. Vibrators offer most of their stimulation through vibrating and come in different shapes and sizes. Some of them are customized on the client's preference, making them diverse and multipurpose. Anal vibrators are meant for anal insertion while bullet ones are inserted in the vagina and may incorporate a finger or a cock ring. The curved G-spot vibrators are curved to access the woman's G-spot.

- Nipple Toys- These are toys meant to stimulate the nipples through their sensitive material and shape. Some may need a varying degree of pressure to be effective while others, such as suction devices, use glass or rubber. They apply to a woman or a man with the use of other toys in other body parts.

    - Penile Toys- These toys are meant to cause stimulation to the penis. For example, the pocket pussies or the artificial vaginas are tubes made of soft tissues to make it feel like a real vagina. A variation of the device may incorporate a system similar to that of a milking machine. A cock harness is used to maintain erection and is worn around the penis. Similarly, cock rings are used to hold the blood in the penis to maintain an erection and may have a clitoris stimulator to perform its duty during sex. The cock rings may also vibrate to ensure that both partners get the best from the toy. A sleeve is a cylindrical device that is open on both ends and could be used to form mutual masturbation. There is also a penis extension that is hollow and shorter than a dildo. They are worn on the tip of the penis to achieve deep penetration. It is advisable to wear a condom to hold the toy from falling off.

Factors to Consider When Selecting Sex Toys

Sex toys are becoming popular, especially among the youth and couples. While there are different types of sex toys, some could be exciting and others intimidating. It would be very tricky trying out a toy that you have never used before. For that reason, you should make the following considerations to get the best toy for you and maximize enjoyment and pleasure.

1. Start easy- When selecting your first sex toy, you should start with the simplest toys there is. This way, you can work up to more advanced toys in the future. Start steadily to avoid disappointments and intimidations.

2. Cleanliness- It is essential to keep your body clean and hygienic, especially your genitals. Therefore, ensure you select sex toys that are cleaned easily and less likely to attract bacteria while in storage.

3. Preference- It is common to find that what works for the service provider is not what will work for you. For that reason, you should ensure you acquire a sex toy depending on your likes and preference.

4. Research- Finding reviewed products online has become simpler; hence, the importance of understanding a sex toy before purchasing or trying it.

5. Storage- Extra care is needed when storing sex toys. They could react to materials placed near them. It is common to find silicone or latex toys looking melted.

6. Consult with your partner- It is for your good to be upfront, open, and honest to your partner about the desires you have with sex toys. Similarly, let them know your preference and use their reaction to judge whether they are okay with it.

7. Maintain Communication- It is the most crucial part of sex, especially when using sex toys. This way, your partner lets you know the part that is stimulated by the toy making it possible to discover additional erogenous zones.

8. Maintain Safety- It is advisable to use these toys for the sole purpose for which they are meant. You should be

cautious when using these toys for good sex. Notably, problems occur whenever users fail to follow instructions.

Various Uses of Sex Toys

- Normalize Sensitivity- Partner may have difficulties having intercourse due to their bodies being hypersensitive. It is a common scenario among new couples. Their genitals may not be exposed to sex before and require preparations for the real act. Sex toys could be used slightly to stimulate the genitals, and they will be ready to have sex with time.

- Foreplay- Sex toys are best in causing stimulations, especially for couples, for they are multipurpose and continuous. Partners could use the different types of toys to stimulate each other before they engage in actual sex. It would work miracles for less physically fit couples. It also saves time that partners could take to achieve stimulation.

- Maintain Stimulation- Sex toys do not disappoint when incorporated in sex. They may be used to cause stimulation to both partners having sex more pleasurable. When using sex positions that have limited caressing and kissing, sex toys could be the ultimate solution.

- Prolong Stimulation- In this case, the partners wish to prolong the stimulation even after orgasm and sex. As they relax after sex, couples could continue using the toys to make the stimulation last longer. It could work for men with erectile dysfunction for it aids in a prolonged erection.

- Third Partner- Sex toys could be used in case one of the partners has passed out or cannot reach certain sensitive areas. For instance, a partner would prefer concurrent stimulation on both the anus and the vagina. The sex toys would take one responsibility as the partner handles the other.

With all these uses, you are sure to find the best sex toy that will work for you and your partner. There are few evitable cons of sex toys while the pros make them a must use.

Pros of Sext Toys

1. Enhances Body Knowledge- The use of sex toys during sex helps partners explore each other bodies and understand the part with more sensory stimulation.

2. Enhances Sexual Pleasure- The combination of these toys with sex provides additional pleasure.

3. Self Confidence- While using sex toys, you are sure that sexual stimulation is guaranteed making you aim at attaining satisfaction.

4. Quick Orgasm- The hyper intensive stimulation caused by sex toys reduces the time a partner would require attaining an orgasm. For that reason, sex starts at the right time with little effort applied.

5. Control Sexual Needs- Sex toys could be used by either partner for sexual stimulation.

6. Fosters Love- The exploration of your partner's genitals as well as communication as you try out sex toys removes barriers and enhances mutual connections.

7. Prevents STIs- The use of sex toys means that genitals may not need to make contact thus preventing the spread of sexually transmitted Infections.

8. Improves Performance- The sensitivity associated with sex toys boosts the partner's morale, making them perform above par.

9. Prevents Unwanted Pregnancy- The fact that sex toys do not ejaculate makes it safe for the woman from impregnation.

Cons

1. Toxicity- Materials used to have sex toys may be toxic to your body although few severe cases have come up.

2. Infections- Untidy and contaminated devices may carry bacteria that may end up infecting your body. For that reason, you should ensure that your sex toys are kept safely in a clean environment.

Sex Positions to Overcome Anxiety and Insecurity

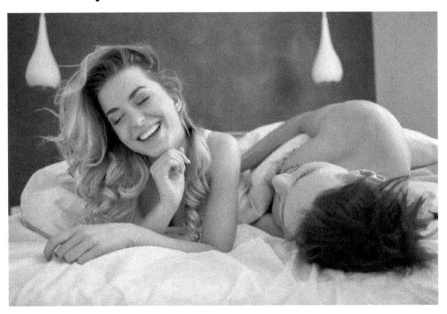

For many people, sex is a natural and easy thing. However, some people have a hard time enjoying it due to the fact that they are insecure. This could be insecurities with their level of experience or with their bodies. In addition, anxiety can truly ruin a mood. It can make it so that one or both parties are unable to reach orgasm. Premature ejaculation can also be a problem in many relationships. Here, we are going to review different positions that can combat all of these negative aspects. With the right positioning, sex can become truly enjoyable without insecurity, anxiety, or the worry of reaching orgasm too soon.

Feeling insecure during sex can make it extremely difficult for you to reach orgasm. Obviously, come with a more relaxed and confident we are the more successful are sex adventures can be. So, finding some positions where you feel truly comfortable is advantageous, especially when you're feeling a bit insecure.

Having sex in a chair is a great position when you are feeling a bit insecure. The man will sit in the chair and the female will simply straddle their legs while facing them. It will allow the person on top to move up and down and grinding will also be possible. This is a very close and intimate position. It will make you feel secure because you'll be facing the person you trust, and your bodies will be tightly wrapped together. It is quite reassuring and will also allow you guys to communicate through the session when you need too.

One other great position is going to happen when both parties are laying on their sides and facing each other. To do this is very simple. The female will need to be slightly higher than the male counterpart. She will have one leg outstretched and one leg draped over his hips. He will then be able to move him closely for insertion. Both parties will be able to move their hips and get a nice rocking motion happening. It allows people to feel extremely secure because you are close enough to talk, kiss, caress each other, and make eye contact. Your bodies will be touching each other completely. It helps both parties feel comfortable and secure.

Basically, any sex position that allows you to face your partner and puts the majority of your body into contact with yours is going to help you feel less insecure. Eye contact is extremely important. In addition, the ability to kiss and caress your partner is also important. So, when you are looking for positions that will reduce your insecurity it is best to choose ones where you are facing one another.

Having anxiety about sex is not uncommon. Unfortunately, many people feel this way from time to time. There are a variety of different sex positions that you can enter into that will help reduce the level of anxiety that you are experiencing. Obviously, being open and communicating with your partner about the fact that you're feeling anxious is a key element in helping you release this negative feeling.

The first position that you should try is commonly referred to as the connected hearts. This is very similar to the cowgirl style. The difference is instead of the man lying flat on his back he will prop himself up with his arms. This will allow you guys to come into contact with one another as the woman rides the man. Your eyes will be able to lock, and you will easily be able to cross each other's bodies. It also will provide you with a good amount of eye contact. This can be pretty intense. If you find that this position increases your anxiety turn the female around so that her back is facing her partner.

Doggie style is another great position when you're feeling anxiety. It allows for a good amount of contact, but you won't have to look each other in the face. Sometimes, staring at your partner in the eyes can be too intense an increase in the level of anxiety that you are experiencing. Doggie style puts both people in control but allows for a higher level of comfort. The view for the man is very nice and the woman has the ability to concentrate on the sensations at hand rather than the intimacy that can come when facing your partner.

Premature ejaculation can be a serious worry for a lot of men. When you are experiencing sexual interaction the last thing you want to do is blow your load too early. It can become such a bother that it negatively impacts a man's performance. Many people don't know that there are a variety of different positions that you can try that can help slow down premature ejaculation. Let's take a few moments and look at some different positions that can help you last longer and ensure that you have what it takes to get your lady to the point of climax.

Any position that has the female on top is fantastic in helping delay premature ejaculation. It can be performed while sitting up or laying down, it really is up to whatever is most comfortable for both of you. She will be able to control what is happening. The man will have some motion that he can add but it really will be up to the woman. This will allow her to decide when it is time for him to have an orgasm. When she realizes that he is almost there, she can completely remove herself from his member or change the speed at which she is moving. This is excellent in helping to control when the man's orgasm will occur.

Side-by-side sex positions are also fantastic in controlling premature ejaculation. This is due to the fact that you will not be able to get as deep during penetration. To accomplish this both parties will lay on their side and the man will position his body between the woman's legs.

The tighter she holds her legs together the less insertion he will be able to accomplish. Both parties will be able to move but there will not be as much movement as with positions such as doggie style. When you are trying to last for a good amount of time this is a position that will be advantageous.

The spooning position is another great one when trying to hinder premature ejaculation. It is also a position where you are on your side so it limits the amount of penetration that you can accomplish. Basically, any position that will not allow you to thrust hard and fast or accomplish an extremely deep level of penetration is going to help you Ward off a fast orgasm.

It is important to note that premature ejaculation is typically more of a burden for the man than it is for a woman. If you do find that you suffer from this issue, there are not only sex positions to help you but there are other things you can do to ensure that your partner is satisfied. If you reach orgasm more quickly than you would prefer it doesn't mean that your sex session has to end. It may be a bit messy but fingering your lady after you have reached climax inside of her can be truly erotic. It can allow her to reach orgasm without you needing to worry about the fact that you ejaculated fairly quickly.

While we like to provide you with sex positions that will help you, we also should warn you that there are some that you should avoid. Doggie style, in particular, is a position that you will not want to enter into if premature ejaculation is a problem. Not only is the view from behind extremely arousing to a man the level of control is, as well. Doggie style allows for extremely deep levels of penetration and movements that can be hard and fast. Hard fast movements combined with deep levels of penetration are guaranteed to make a man ejaculate quickly. So, if you are trying to avoid a quick climax you should avoid this position at all costs.

Keep in mind, that we've only given you a look at the variety of different sex positions that can help with insecurity, anxiety, and premature ejaculation. If none of these seem to be working for you do a bit more research and try some new things. You never know what that is out there will work better than the guidance that we have provided. However, most people find great success in the positions that we have provided, and it leads them to more fulfilling sex life. This goes for not only you but also for your partner.

Easy Tips to Make Her Hornier and Spicing Up your Sex life

A standout amongst the most successive protestations men have about their spouses is that they wish their ladies would start sex all the more frequently, or if nothing else that they would be more receptive to their sexual suggestions. The explanation behind this basic inconsistency is that male sexual yearning is heartier and more unconstrained, while female sexual craving is more variable and receptive to the earth.

With regards to sex, men are for the most part genitally centered, while for ladies, sex is a full psyche and body experience. The fundamental clash between men furthermore, ladies, sexually, is that men are similar to firefighters, and ladies are similar to flame. To men, sex is a crisis, and regardless of what they're doing, they can be prepared in two minutes. Ladies, then again, are similar to flame. They're extremely energizing, yet the conditions have to be precisely a good fit for it to happen.

FOR WOMEN TO WANT SEX IT HAS TO BE SEX WORTH HAVING.

Therefore, to sexually motivate her, you have to really work on having sex so exciting for her so that she considers it a priority.

- Attempt Mellow Subjugation And/Or Discipline

For a few ladies, the considered surrendering obligation regarding their sexual fulfillment is an intense turn-on. Set her up by advising her what you will do to her this evening (you can leave her a note or a voice message or send her an email). Request that she get ready for it by wearing your top pick "slave" outfit and making herself lovely. At the point when the time comes, arrange her to get down on her knees and submit to her "expert."

Tie her tenderly with a delicate servitude thing, which can likewise be utilized to gently tease her areolas. You can then continue to tease her with a plume or a tickler or give her a light punishing with your hand. Sex toys can likewise be utilized here.

Keep in mind: The object of the overwhelming/docile diversion is not mortification or torment; it is to convey her to peak, and conceivably more than once.

- Attempt Role Playing

Imagine you are a Penthouse picture taker and welcome her to posture for you, or a pizza conveyance fellow who really likes her, or a policeman capturing her as she is about to escape her auto. This is another variation of investigating her dreams (and yours).

One awesome approach to enjoy what is likely a common dream is to request that her play a stripper or a call young lady with you as her supporter. On the off chance that she appreciates performing for you, you can indeed, even make your own grown-up video and replay it together later on. You would be shocked at what number of ladies fantasize about being in such suggestive parts - just social strictures keep them from letting it be known.

In our general public, which quietly underwrites and advances the Madonna/prostitute dichotomy, giving her consent to showcase her "skanky" dreams or requesting her to "be awful" may very well draw out that skank that you have been longing to have in your room.

- Empower Her Sexual Care

Numerous ladies don't get stirred in light of the fact that their brain floats off as opposed to concentrating on the sensuality existing apart from everything else. To direct her musings far from that shopping rundown and to keep her "careful," get her front of the mirror and advise her to watch what you are going to do to her. Verbally depicting every demonstration of foreplay before you do it is additionally a method for keeping her psyche on the warmth existing apart from everything else. Begin by kissing her neck and shoulders as you rub your hands on her dressed body.

84

At that point, gradually evacuate her underwear yet leave whatever is left of her garments on. Lift her shirt or dress and delicately touch her areolas as you rub her base. Sit her on a seat before the mirror and request her to touch her vulva. You can even request that she rubs some genital warming oil like Zestra on her vaginal lips while you watch. Direct her hands as you inquire her to perform a self-excitement. On the other hand, motivate her to portray her sensations with every move you make. Before long, she will be imploring you to have intercourse with her.

- Search her fantasies

Request that her let you know her dreams or to email them to you. Urge her to depict them in point of interest. The closeness that such an admission produces will be sexually stirring for her. Be that as it may, be arranged for the unforeseen. In the event that she reveals that the considered being with another lady (or Brad Pitt) turns her on, don't get bothered or unstable. Rather, misuse it further bolstering your good fortune. While you are kissing and stroking her, turn a storyline that matches her dream. Whisper it in her ear and let her toll in with her own points of interest - which you can use to coordinate your lips and hands. In the event that her psyche likens your touch with her most profound dreams, she will begin getting wet at your first stroke.

- Watch Erotica Together

Numerous ladies lean toward aural to visual erotica. Have a go at perusing a hot short story together. Pick one where the "activity" suits your wishes, as well, and read it to her. With regards to visual erotica, numerous ladies lean toward materials that have a plot, and that stress enthusiasm and association between the heroes. That implies leaving your most loved butt-centric bash DVD for your private autoerotic sessions. Rather, watch a hot adults-only film, for example, 9 1/2 Weeks, or buy an X-appraised video with a storyline by Candida Royalle.

- Use Verbal Support

In our general public, which venerates ceaseless youth and frequently sets impossible magnificence models, numerous ladies feel unreliable about their looks and hesitant about their bare bodies. At the point when a lady feels unreliable, she is unrealistic to be in the state of mind for sex. To build her sexual responsiveness, advise her in the middle of kisses and as you touch her body that you locate her excellent and provocative, that she turns you on and that you need to appreciate all aspects of her body before having intercourse to her.

Pay her some particular compliments - advise her you adore her comforting grin, her delicate skin or the shape, size and feel of her bosoms. What's more, don't sit tight for sexual minutes to run out such verbal fortifications.

- Be a good Kisser

To be a specialist kisser, begin delicately and work up to more enthusiasm in slow stages. Start by scarcely brushing your lips against hers, and after that touch her lips with the tip of your tongue. Unwind and open your lips as you develop the kiss, yet abstain from dribbling, drooling then again overwhelming vacuum sucking.

On the off chance that you are stressed over terrible breath, make sure to brush your tongue and your teeth, particularly on the off chance that you have been drinking espresso or smoking. In the event that you can't brush, bite on a lemon peel or a mint, or pop a self-dissolving oral consideration strip into your mouth sometime recently starting. You can likewise apply lip medicine with menthol or mint and delicately rub your lips against your accomplices to share the shiver. Take a stab at keeping eye contact by not shutting your eyes while you kiss. For some ladies, this extends the association and supercharges their sex drive.

Be More Arousing in Your Touches

A greater part of lady's incline toward delicate, delicate touches and strokes everywhere on their body until they get completely stimulated. Sex advisors call this kind of touch "non-interest touch" or "delight centered outer course." Don't simply snatch her bosoms or butt; rather, let your hands gradually achieve those objectives with long, tender touches. When she is completely excited and dribbling with craving, she may love the rougher play, however, save that Neanderthal beast in you for the real intercourse.

- Lengthen the foreplay

The old cliché is true: Ladies love foreplay. Foreplay does not mean quickly getting her clitoris. Genuine foreplay means beginning as a long way from her private parts as would be prudent - holding her face, stroking her hair, kissing her sanctuaries, looking at her, or rubbing her neck and shoulders. Realize some back-rub systems and delicately attempt a couple on her head, neck and shoulders.

Work your direction southward gradually. Take a stab at utilizing only the light touch of your fingertips called pattes d'araignee (the English interpretation "bug legs" some way or another invokes the wrong picture).

- Improve the environment

We now and again experience issues blocking boisterously commotions like you're yapping pooch or booming television lights or disregarding the harmful odors of spoiled nourishment exuding from your untidy kitchen. Yes, that implies killing the TV, darkening the lights, encouraging your pooch, turning up your indoor regulator, taking out the trash and washing the filthy bed covers. In the event that the idea of doing this discourages your sex drive, employ a housekeeper.

Spicing up your sex life

Learning how to spice up your sex life is something every couple should do. Even if things seem to be going on just well, they can always be better. You can never have enough of your partner. Spicing means trying new stuff or doing things differently. One of the ways to spice our sex life is by learning new sex positions. They always add some freshness and the process of trying them out is so much fun.

- Sexual fetishes

Fetishes are using body parts, objects or materials to lead up to an elevated state of sexual arousal. They may also be referred to as sexual preferences or kinks. These enhance the sexual experiences in a manner that normal sex wouldn't. For couples, it can be a good way to improve your sex life. Talking about sexual fetishes with your partner and actually trying them out can lead to deep sexual satisfaction. The key here is to talk about it as some fetishes might cross your partner's boundaries. However, if it does no harm, doesn't compromise one's beliefs and is legal, then there shouldn't be a reason not to try it out. Keep in mind that the fetish doesn't have to be performed each time you indulge in sex rather occasionally to heighten the pleasure. In fact, a fetish doesn't always need to be performed; even talking about it can bring so much pleasure to some people. Exploring each other fetishes means you are both very comfortable with other and intimately close. You can initiate the conversation with your partner regarding anything special that they'd like to try out in the bedroom.

- Talking dirty to your partner

Is there anybody who doesn't love some dirty talk from their partner? I doubt there is. Dirty talk is one way in which couples can bring back the oomph to their sex life. Couples should seize every opportunity available to tell each other how much they want them and what they need them to do. Even if the situation doesn't allow you to jump into each other's arms, you'll slowly build the anticipation and by the time you hit the sack, everything will just be waiting to explode. When having sex, always talk with your partner and let them know how they make you feel. Men, in particular, are turned on by dirty talking during sex. Women, on the other hand, love dirty talk before sex to bring them to the mood. You can send each other sexy sex messages during the day. You don't have to be very creative with words. Just a simple phrase lets your partner knows you are thinking about them and you can't wait to have them.

It might seem awkward to initiate dirty talk if you haven't been doing it before but it's worth it. Just try it maybe at first using a text message before you say it to your partner. These small things make all the difference.

- Rekindling romance

After the initial excitement fizzles out, it is possible to get into a rut. Rekindling romance improves our sex life as well. Romance and sex go hand in hand. However, we shouldn't confuse sex for romance, like most men are likely to do. But when a partner feels loved and appreciated, they open up more leading to better sex. Without romance, our sex lives are the first to suffer. We might find ourselves just going through the motions without really achieving much emotionally. Romance can be rekindled by expressing your desire for your partner and appreciating them. Go out for dates every once in a while, and always make an effort to please your partner. If you have kids, take some time when you can have someone look after them and just enjoy each other's company with no distractions at all. Plan for a honeymoon vacation every year to reconnect with your partner is another option. Our professional lives can eat up so much of our time that we lose the connection with our partner. Talk with your partner daily not just about the kids or the finances but also about yourselves. This makes you know your partner more and understand them. Believe me, even people married for decades have something new to learn about their partner. Engaging in a new activity can help you spend more time together. You might pick a new hobby, pick an exercise plan or just make a point of going out more often. All these will translate to a better sex life due to the increased intimacy and connection.

- Spontaneous vs. scheduled sex

We plan everything important in life be it meetings, doctor's appointments, meeting with friends and anything else in between. But when it comes to sex, most of us cringe at the idea of scheduling sex. Spontaneous sex is the best, everybody agrees, but our busy schedules often don't allow time for it. People are working more and more hours. Partners can often feel like roommates when their schedules crash or one of them is too tired or not in the mood. This is where setting aside time for sex can really play an important role. At this time, sex is the number one priority, it's the only thing. Everything else is set aside and we focus on making love. Younger lovers might find this idea not quite appealing, but it can help if you find yourselves having no time for sex.

However, scheduling sex doesn't mean you can't have the spontaneous sex when possible. In fact, you should also plan for spontaneity. This is by having in place anything you require for sex at the right place for when you have sex. If you use condoms or lubricants, realizing just before you have sex that you don't have any left can be quite a disappointment.

BDSM

Introduction/ What is it?

BDSM stands for Bondage, Discipline, Dominant and Submissive, Sadism and Masochism. The four letters in this acronym overlap and form a large umbrella term that encompasses a wide variety of practices, preferences, kinks and fetishes of a sexual nature. Under this umbrella, there is something for everyone no matter what you enjoy sexually and probably many things that you didn't even know existed that would turn you on if you explored them. Everything included in BDSM comes down to finding pleasure and being open to experiences and practices that may not be considered the "norm" in society. It is about finding these things and accepting these parts of yourself and other people without restrictions or judgment. Entering the world of BDSM will give you a space to allow yourself to explore a different world and find out what makes you feel good in the bedroom by yourself as well as with one or multiple partners.

Bondage

Bondage is the act of tying up or restraining a partner during sex. The restricted movement that this causes makes people feel sexually aroused because they are unable to move, and as a result their sexual desire builds and builds. As it builds and they want to touch themselves they are unable to do so, which means they are unable to help themselves find release by either touching their own genitals (to give themselves an orgasm), or by touching their partner who is freely moving and can touch themselves or the person that is restrained. Sometimes, the person who is not restrained will tease the person they have tied up or handcuffed by touching themselves or touching the other person but not enough to actually make them orgasm. This makes the restrained person become very sexually frustrated to the point where they want to rip off whatever is restraining them. The fact that they can't makes them even more frustrated and thus aroused.

When they are finally allowed to move, whether they touch themselves, have penetrative sex with their partner or their partner gives them an orgasm in some other way, it makes for a mind-blowing orgasm because their pent-up pleasure and sexual tension has been finally released.

For the person who enjoys restraining their partner during sex, having control is usually the reason why this brings them pleasure. Because they are tying up or handcuffing their partner, they also get to decide when to release their partner. This gives them a sense of power and control over someone else which can make people feel very sexually aroused. The part that makes this bring a person sexual pleasure is that their partner is usually naked and quite aroused- meaning they have an erection or are quite wet if they have a vagina. The restrained person may be begging them to touch their genitals or do something sexual to them, but the partner in control has the power to decide when and if they will do this. They then have full control over the pleasure of their partner. They get to decide what they want to do and how they want to do it, which gives them a sense of excitement and this is a turn-on sexually.

- Discipline

Discipline comes into play during bondage when the person who is tied up, handcuffed or restrained in some other way gets disciplined. This discipline can be in the form of being spanked or whipped or some type of physical discipline such as this while practicing bondage. Discipline can also be of a psychological nature. This is done by using psychological restraint such as Edging or having to hold back in any sense (such as being silent). Some people become sexually aroused by having to hold back in any sense whether it be holding back an orgasm, holding back moans of pleasure, holding back from touching your partner or anything of the sort. This can be combined with physical discipline where if the person cannot or chooses not to hold themselves back, they will be disciplined by being spanked or whipped. The looming threat of being disciplined is a turn-on to those who enjoy being afraid play into their sex life.

- Dominant

Dominance is a practice within BDSM that is more of a mental practice, but it can take a physical form as well in the bedroom. For example, in the sects of BDSM that we have looked at already (bondage and discipline) there is a person who ties their partner up or who spanks their partner. This person who is doing the tying or the restricting of some sort is usually the dominant partner. This person could be referred to as the "Dom." This person becomes sexually aroused by being in control or in a position of power and by having their partner give up all control to them. they become aroused by knowing that their partner must submit to them and must ask them if they want or need something. Usually, this practice of being dominant will be combined with other aspects of BDSM like the two examples I gave.

- Submissive

Submission is also a practice within BDSM and is on the flip side of the Dominance coin. In a sexual relationship where there is a Dom, there will likely be a Sub as well. The submissive partner becomes sexually aroused by being tied up, being spanked and/ or having to ask their Dominant partner for what they want. They become aroused by giving up total control of their pleasure to the other person. When in a submissive position sexually, they have no choice but to let their pleasure take over their body, and when it reaches an extreme level, they are unable to do anything about it without first asking the other person or having the other person do it for them. For example, touching them or releasing them so that they can touch themselves. The pent-up pleasure makes for an intense orgasm when it is finally released, and this is why some people enjoy either mentally holding back by submitting to psychological discipline or being physically forced to hold back. Usually, you will see this position, or this person referred to as the Sub.

S&M

Sadism and masochism, commonly known as S&M, is the addition of pain play into your sexual experiences. The thin line between pleasure and pain is ridden here to give extreme pleasure mixed with a little bit of fear. The Dominance and Submission roles that we just discussed come into practice here as well as there will be someone who is inflicting pain and someone who would be the receiver of pain- usually the Dom and the Sub, respectively.

- Sadist

A sadist is a person who gets pleasure from inflicting pain on another. Within BDSM, this is in a sexual context. This person becomes sexually aroused and excited by inflicting pain on their partner. This practice actually comes down to being turned on by the power that they have when they are in charge of inflicting pain. This is similar to the Dominant person in a Dom/Sub relationship, where the dominant partner is aroused by having the power of being in control.

- Masochist

A masochist is a person who gets pleasure from being in pain at the hands of their partner. This person gets sexual pleasure from riding the line between pleasure and pain. This is similar to the Submissive role in a Dom/Sub relationship. This person enjoys giving up the power to their partner and being unable to take control of their own body or their own sexual experience.

BDSM Sex Positions

As you can see now, most of these sections within BDSM are overlapping with others, and there is some grey area as to where one begins and the other ends. All or any of these can be combined in a single sexual encounter or with a specific couple, or they could occur on their own. The decision is up to the couple themselves about what they are comfortable including in their sex life and what they want to leave out.

We will now continue our exploration of sex positions by looking at some different sex positions that fall into these above categories and therefore under the general umbrella that is BDSM. This will give you a more specific idea of what types of sex positions are considered BDSM, what this would look like in practice and where to start if you want to experiment with BDSM a little bit. Many of these positions we will look at will involve the overlap of a few of the seven terms explained above, it is difficult to separate many of them which is why they all come together to form the all-encompassing term that is BDSM.

- Blindfolded Massage

Sensory Deprivation is a type of bondage that is a great place to start if you are just dabbling in the world of BDSM. You can use anything as a blindfold, and the different things you use can really add to the experience. Try using one of your ties, or an item of the woman's clothing to add to the heat of the moment factor.

Imagine you just got home from a long day at work and on your drive home, you were thinking about how you can't wait to have sex with your wife, getting yourself all hot and bothered the entire drive. You get home and she is also horny, waiting for you to arrive so she can rip off your clothes. When the time comes that you want to add in the element of restriction, tell her to close her eyes. Untie your tie from your neck and wrap it around her eyes slowly. Whisper in her ear while you do this and watch all of her other senses heighten as her vision is gone. From here, you can touch her lightly and her skin all over will be much more sensitive than it normally is. To spice this encounter up, even more, grab things like a feather duster, silk sheets, or anything with texture. Gently glide the feather duster down her back or over her breasts and the sensations will overwhelm her. Once her body is on high alert and feeling everything much stronger, you can begin with a massage of her breasts and eventually, her clitoris. If you want to keep going you can then have sex with the blindfold on too, or you can throw it off and switch gears entirely but after this blindfolded massage she is sure to be sensitive all over and ready for a very intense orgasm.

- Handcuffs/Tying Up

Handcuffs are a sexy and simple introduction to the world of restraint and domination, that you have probably heard of before. This is a great place to start because the person being restricted can still express their desires and wishes for pleasure, but the other person is ultimately in charge of what they choose to agree to and what they do not. Because both partners can still see and talk to each other, they can communicate throughout, telling the other person how to touch them and what they like. The fact that one partner is in control will be the thing that makes both of you go wild with desire.

- Restrained Eagle

Begin with your partner lying down on their back and handcuff their hands to the bed frame, spread out from each other at a comfortable distance. From here, you can give them oral pleasure, or you can rub their genitals with your hands. If you want to drive them crazy, you can tease them from afar. Start touching yourself in front of them, telling them how good it feels and how much you like it, knowing that they cannot do anything. Thinking of all the things they would like to do to you and the places they would like to touch you and themselves will make them so horny they will barely be able to contain it. This position is great for dirty talk as well.

You can take this position any direction you like after this, but the point is that teasing your partner and being in control of touching them and touching yourself will have them so pleasurably frustrated. You can proceed to penetration in this position as well if that turns both of you on, with you taking full control of their pleasure.

- Rope Tied Kneeling

If you have tried using handcuffs and would like to take it a little further and want to experiment with a bit more submission, you can try adding an element of role-playing into your restraint by using rope instead of the soft and fluffy handcuffs you can buy at a sex shop. Using rope will make it feel a bit more risqué and much different from the ultra-safe feeling you will get from handcuffs bought from a sex shop. Don't get me wrong, these handcuffs can be fun too, but if you want to take it to the next level you can use something a little barer bone. Feeling like you used whatever you had handy can make you both feel like you are doing something secret and, in the moment, and the thrill of spontaneity always comes with some excitement-induced arousal.

Kneel at the top of the bed facing the bed frame with your hands together on top of it. Have your man come up behind you and reach around to tie your wrists to the bed frame. Using rope will make it feel a bit more frightening and if you are looking for the next step up from handcuffs, this is it. From your restrained position here, tell him to slide his penis into you from behind and begin thrusting. All you will be able to do is tell him what you want and what you like, but you cannot touch him or yourself, so your pleasure relies on his touch.

- Biting

Want to try a little bit of pain play? While you must try this with a partner you trust in order to have the best experience possible, a bit of biting is a good place to start exploring the world of S&M.

- Vampire Missionary

You can try this position any time as an entry to some of the different types of sexual pain-pleasure that are commonly practiced. You can try this having discussed it beforehand with your partner, or if you prefer you can spring it on them at the moment and see how they react. Doing it surprisingly in the moment this way could lead to an unexpected surge in lust as they may not even know that they are turned on by being bitten during sex. When trying to introduce a new type of play into your sex life, doing it in a sexual position you are familiar with will allow you to focus on the new things going on instead of trying to also figure out how to get into a complicated position. To introduce biting or pain play into your sex, try it for the first time in the Missionary position so that you are comfortable and close to your partner so that you both can communicate easily with each other throughout.

While your man is on top of you in the Missionary Position with his face close to yours, turn your head and kiss his neck gently. Begin to lightly suck on his neck skin and get him used to your mouth being around this area. The skin on the neck is very thin and sensitive and that is why so many people enjoy being kissed there. When he is already enjoying this, you can progress to the next stage. The next step is to introduce a little bit of a bite on his ultra-sensitive neck skin. See if he likes this. He may even like the idea so much that he gets into it and starts to do it back to you. If so, you can feel it out and see if it is something that you like having done to you too. Then, as your sex heats up, gently bite his shoulder as he is thrusting into you. While you are making out, you can slowly nibble on his lip to add a little bit of a power dynamic and a bit of pain into the steamy moment.

Flirting and Courtship

Flirting and courtship are two very important aspects of any relationship, as without them we would never be able to woo our partner and attract them to us. We all have our own unique style of flirting, some of us being better at it than others, but thankfully the Kama Sutra lays out exactly what we should be doing in order to be the best flirter possible.

Before we dive into the art of courtship and the tricks to up your flirting game, we will break down exactly what flirting and courtship are and how they differ. Flirting is something that is done with a less serious intention in mind than when you court someone. Flirting can be both sexual as well as friendly, and people can engage in it for fun just as much as they can use it to attract a partner. Typically flirting involves using both verbal and non-verbal communication in order to let someone know that you are interested in them. It can involve a wink, touching someone's arm, laughing at their jokes, or any other of ways in which you showcase your interest.

Courting, on the other hand, is more serious in nature and it is dating someone with the intention of marrying them. Some religious beliefs feel that the only acceptable form of dating is courting, while others engage in courting, not for religious reasons but because they are simply at a point in life where they are looking to get married. Courting can, and should, involve flirting, but it is used to win the other person over and entice them to want to marry you. It is never simply used to instigate a fling or sexual encounter, as that would be in direct contradiction to the point of courting.

Now that we have a basic understanding of the two terms, what exactly does the Kama Sutra say when it comes to courting and flirting?

Meeting the Person, You Want to Date

To begin with, the Kama Sutra starts by mentioning that anyone looking to court another should be realistic in their approach. What this means is that any quality that they are seeking in another, they should possess that quality themselves otherwise they have no right to expect it of their partner. For instance, if you want your partner to be extremely good looking, you yourself should also be extremely good looking otherwise you should not put such a demand on someone else. Once you have your expectations in check, then you can begin the processes of searching for your partner.

So, how does one go about seeking out a woman in ancient times when there was no social media and no dating apps? Well, the Kama Sutra suggests the following ways:

- A woman who is ready to be married should be dressed up nicely by her family and placed in a location where she can be seen

- Women seeking a husband should attend events such as sporting matches and marriage ceremonies

- Men should throw parties in which games are played, causing everyone to interact with each other

- Through friendships, two people can then meet and get to know each other

- By asking their parents, a man can have a wife arranged for him

Of course, we can add much more to this list for current times, so if you are at the point in your life where you are looking to meet someone and build towards marriage, or a future in general, you can try the following more common suggestions as well:

- Try going online and joining a dating site - Nowadays there are numerous different sites, all catering to different individuals and desires, so you are likely to find a site that is perfect for you and finding a partner that matches what you are after

- Ask your friends to hook you up with someone - We know the idea of going on a blind date sounds terrifying, but your friends do know you well, so there is always the chance that they might know someone who fits in with what you are looking for

- Participate in a sport or hobby – Take up a new activity that interests you in order to meet new people and also meet someone who shares similar interests with you. Not only will you already have something to talk about, but it gets you out of the house and on a mini date right from day one

- Take the bus to work – While your morning commute is never fun, why not turn it into an opportunity to meet someone? Public transportation puts you in close proximity with new people that you have never met before

However, you choose to approach meeting someone, that is only the first step in courtship, as the real work is what comes afterward.

Beginning a Courtship

Once you have found an individual who interests you, who you would like to get closer with and possibly start a relationship, how are you supposed to let them know that you are interested? In modern times, we have many ways of determining if someone is interested in us, and many of these various ways full under the heading of flirting. When we are attracted to someone, either physically or mentally, or both, our bodies automatically respond to them in specific ways. Some of what we do is deliberate, while other actions are completely subconscious and are naturally done simply because we want to be near someone.

Some of the common ways of flirting that you may be more familiar with are:

- Making direct eye contact
- Holding eye contact longer than normal
- Smiling when you look at a person
- Touching them on the arm when you talk
- Winking from across a room
- Complimenting the other person
- Biting of the lip
- Playing with your hair
- Mirroring another person's movements
- Laugh at their silly jokes
- Stand closely
- Stare at their lips
- Keep your arms uncrossed and open
- Tease them playfully
- Drop a witty pick-up line
- Send a flirtatious text message

Sadly, you won't find any of these located within the Kama Sutra as back in ancient India flirting and courting were done much differently. To compare with the above list, let's take a look at different ways in which the Kama Sutra suggests a man flirts with a woman to show her that he is interested and to engage her attention:

- Spend time with her and entertain her with games

- Pick flowers and turn them into a garland

- Cook meals together

- Play with dice or cards

- Playgroup games such as hide and seek

- Do gymnastic exercises together

- Show kindness to her friends

- Partake in services for her maid's daughter to win her over

- Get her gifts that no other girls have

- Give her handmade dolls and wooden figures

- Create temples for her dedicated to different goddesses

- Make her see him as someone who can do everything for her

- Meet her in private

- Tell her exciting stories

- Perform tricks and juggle

- Sing for her and take her to festivals

- Give her flowers and jewelry

- Teach her nurses daughter the 64 forms of pleasure

While many of these sounds a bit strange in today's time, there is a lot we can take away from this list. Mainly, everything described above is meant to make the man stand out from other men that may have an interest in the same woman. This is exactly what modern-day flirting and courting involves as well, as you want to make the other person see what you have to offer and what they will find in you that they cannot find in someone else. Flirting and courting are meant to entice another person, that is their sole purpose, and to let that person know that you would like to be in a relationship with them, or at the very least engage in some sort of romantic endeavor.

Many people get stressed out by the idea of flirting, and so often you will hear individuals remark that they are unable to flirt or are the worst at doing so. This is simply a false idea that they have gotten into them hear, and they are making it into something much more complicated than it needs to be. Flirting does not need to be anything more than smiling at a person you like or going out of your way to do something nice for them. All you are aiming to do is make them feel special and noticed, and to hopefully get them to notice you in return. The best way to go about it if you lack confidence is to simply start off small. You don't need to perform a magic trick or juggle, and instead you can simply compliment their outfit or send them a text asking about their day. The basic act of taking notice goes a very long way as it shows the person you are thinking of them and that you are interested in who they are. Don't overcomplicate things, and let it progress naturally as you feel more comfortable. Once you get outside of your own head, you will find flirting to be one of the most natural acts possible.

A Woman's State of Mind

Within the Kama Sutra, Vatsyayana goes into detail about a woman's state of mind during flirting and courtship and breaks down the different ways she may feel and react, as well as how many should respond to her. Some of the advice is practical and useful even in today's world, but other tips are much more non-consensual and should not ever be utilized. Here are the mindsets that are mentioned along with the details attributed to each one:

A Woman Who Listens but Does Not Show Any Interest

In this scenario, a man should attempt to persuade her by using a middleman instead of just doing it on his own. A good option would be her nurse's daughter or one of her friends.

If a Woman Meets a Man Once and Then the Next Time Is Better Dressed

This indicates that she is very interested, and thus the man will need to do little in order to win her over. If, however, after a long period of time she still does not consent to be with him, then he should be wary but still keep her as a close friend.

When a Woman Avoids A Man Out of Respect

In this scenario, it will be difficult to win her over, but the man can do so by keeping her as a close friend and also employing the assistance of a very crafty middleman.

If a Woman Turns a Man Down Harshly

When this happens, a man should abandon his attempts to win her over and move on to someone else, for she had no interest in anything he has to offer her.

When Meeting Privately She Allows His Touch but Pretends Not to Notice

If this happens then it means she is interested but playing coy, so he should continue on with his advances. It will require extra patience, but he can begin by putting his arm around her while she sleeps and seeing how she reacts. If it is a favorable reaction, then he can continue on by drawing her closer to him and continuing on from there.

If a Woman Does Not Encourage nor Discourage a Man's Advances, but Instead Is Hidden Away in a Place He Cannot Get To

The only option in this situation is to employ the help of someone who is close to her in order to communicate his advances. The best option would be the daughter of her maid. If the woman does not respond to the man through the go-between, then he should reconsider whether or not to continue pursuing her.

When A Woman Proclaims Her Own Interest in The Man

If this happens, then the man can know for sure that she is wanting to be with him, and he can delight in enjoying her fully. In order to realize this situation, however, the man must know the ways in which a woman will show her interest. Ways in which a woman will manifest her love towards a man are:

- She speaks to him without being addressed first

- She meets with him in private

- When she talks her voice trembles

- Her hands and feet will perspire

- Her face will blush with delight

- She will shampoo his body and rub his head

- When washing him she only uses one hand, and instead uses the other hand to caress him

- She stands motionless with both hands pressed against him

- She bends down and places her face on his thighs

- If she places her hand upon him, she keeps it there for a long period of time

The most important thing noted when discussing wooing over a woman, however, is how she responds within the first conversation that a man has with her. The Kama Sutra notes that a man must find a way to be introduced to the woman that he is interested in, and from there he can then carry out a conversation to assess her feelings. By subtle means of flirting, he should try and let the woman know that he has love for her, and if she responds to this in a positive way, then he should continue on with pursuing her over time. If the woman is very open to his expressions of love, and outwardly responds in a favorable manner, then he knows he will be able to gain her over as a wife very easily. Finally, if a woman is open enough to express her love back verbally, then the man will know right then and there that she is his. Vatsyayana believed that this was true for all women, regardless of who they are, where they were from, or how they were raised, and in many ways, this still holds true today.

It may all sound like very obvious information, but when our brains are overtaken by feelings of love, our judgment can become clouded and we may miss some of the most obvious signals that someone else is attracted to us as well. That is why it is important to have them written down in a book like the Kama Sutra, so that even in moments of overwhelming desire we are reminded of the simple truths that come with flirting and courting. Mainly, what we are discussing are various aspects of consent, and how pursuing someone who is not interested in us will not get us very far. While the Kama Sutra often encourages a man to keep trying, it specifies that when a woman harshly turns you down, then it is time to leave her be. You should never force yourself on someone else, and in fact, why would you want to? We all want to be loved and desired, and none of us should settle for someone who dislikes us or isn't as invested as we are in them.

While the Kama Sutra may have some outdated views on flirting and courtship, the basic principles are still applicable even after all of the centuries which have passed since it was written. Take the time to show someone you are interested, go the extra mile, make them laugh, and employ the help of a mutual friend if you are shy are unsure. Whatever you choose to do, make sure you enjoy the process as flirting and courting are almost sport like in their nature. This is when new feelings are blossoming, and a different picture of the future will unfold in your mind. The best thing you can do is to lose yourself in those feelings and to simply see where they take you. Not every person you pursue will work out, but eventually, you will find that one person that appreciates what you have to offer and will offer you just as much in return.

Conclusion

Now that we have looked at a variety of different positions, it's time to bring this book back around full circle to where we started. All of these positions can lead to an absolutely mind-blowing orgasm, but there is much more that goes into great sex than just switching up how you do it. In order to truly reap all of the benefits these positions offer, you need to make sure you and your partner are working as a team, both inside and outside of the bedroom.

Teamwork includes things like communicating effectively, build on what each other likes, and building each other up as individuals. All of this takes work on both your parts, but the results you will see make it all worth it. Together you can create a great relationship, and the best sex life possible. One in which you experience the deepest orgasm together, each and every time.

Learn what your partner likes

This may seem obvious, but a lot of people actually fall quite short when it comes to this aspect of sex and relationships in general. If you've had sex with other partners prior, you may carry over a lot of what you learned previously into your current sex life. This is not at all a bad thing, but it is important to remember that every person is different and how one individual like to be touched may not be how your new partner likes it.

In order to truly pleasure you partner, you should simply ask them what they like. Let the describe their favorite parts of sex or share with you some of their intimate spots that you might not know to touch. If you are confident and comfortable, have your partner physically show you how they like it by engaging in a bit of mutual masturbation. Not only is this educational, but it can be very arousing watching your partner touch themselves and it can be a great bit of foreplay.

The more you get to know your partner, both mentally and physically, the more in tune you two will be. Being on the same page ensures that sex is beneficial to both of you, and that each of you are invested in the other person enjoying themselves and leaving each interaction completely satisfied.

Some tips on learning and exploring what your partner likes are:

- Simply ask them during sex if what you are doing feels good

- During sex ask them what they would like you to do or touch

- Have them masturbate in front of you, or with you

- Let your partner initiate sex so you know they are eager

- Stay connected outside of the bedroom, ensuring that communication lines are open, and your partner is comfortable opening up to you

- Encourage your partner without criticizing them

- Watch porn together and each point out what turns you on the most

- Both of you be vocal during sex so you each have an auditory clue of what you like and what you may not be a huge fan of

Build up that confidence

Sex can be a very difficult thing for some people, mainly due to embarrassment and confidence issues. These types of problems can severely hinder a great sexual relationship, so it is vital that you both are working together to build the other person up.

If you were unsure if your partner found you attractive, there is very little chance you would want to then get naked in front of them and open yourself up emotionally and physically. This is actually quite common, however, and many people suffer from body issues where they dislike the way they look. Our job as a partner is to make each other feel great about themselves, and to shower them with compliments so that their self-esteem is raised up. You want your partner to want to show themselves to you, so avoid criticizing their appearance or making comments that may hurt how they feel about themselves.

Building confidence starts outside of the bedroom, with the way you treat your partner as well as how you talk to them and interact in general. If you are always nagging or putting your partner down, it won't matter how sexy you find them because their confidence is going to be lowered and their self-worth may not be where it should be. Instead work on building them up throughout the day, and try things such as:

- Complimenting them on the outfit they are wearing

- Thanking them when they do something around the house

- Pay attention when they are speaking and make them feel important

- Taking a genuine interest in their day

- Telling them how proud of them you are

- Smiling when you see them

- Holding their hand

- Appreciate who they are and tell them what you love about them

- Get rid of the idea of perfectionism, and instead find perfection within the imperfections

By taking the time every day to build up your partner, you will end up having a better relationship, and sex life, as a result. There is no bigger turn on than confidence, and when your partner can truly let go and be themselves in the bedroom then there are bound to be fireworks. A lot of positions require trust, confidence, and high self-esteem in order to master, and as a result that needs to be in place before you begin. If you want your spouse to go wild, they need to know it is a safe place where they are free from judgment and criticism.

CPSIA information can be obtained
at www.ICGtesting.com
Printed in the USA
LVHW080311210221
679537LV00006B/170